PLAB 2 MASTER SERIES
VOLUME TWO
CLINICAL SYSTEMS & EMERGENCIES

Clinical Reasoning, Emergency Recognition and Safe Management Across All Specialties

AMaC A. Mansour and Colleagues

AMaC
A. Mansour and Colleagues
United Kingdom
2026

Copyright

First published 2026.

ISBN (Paperback): 978-1-0667467-2-9 · ISBN (Ebook): 978-1-0667467-3-6

First Edition 2026

Published by AMaC Publishing, United Kingdom

www.amac-medical.com

CAUTION — Medical Disclaimer

The information contained in this book is intended solely for examination preparation purposes. It does not constitute clinical advice, medical guidance, or a substitute for professional medical judgement. The authors and publisher make no representations or warranties of any kind, express or implied, about the completeness, accuracy, or suitability of the information contained herein for clinical practice.

Clinical guidelines, drug doses, and protocols change. Readers must always consult current national guidelines, the British National Formulary (BNF), and senior clinical colleagues before applying any information in patient care.

The authors and publisher accept no liability for any loss, injury, or damage arising from the use of this material in any context other than PLAB 2 examination preparation.

PLAB 2 is a registered examination of the General Medical Council (GMC), United Kingdom. This book is an independent examination preparation resource and is not affiliated with, endorsed by, or produced in association with the GMC.

Dedication

To the doctors who already know the medicine
but were never taught how to show it.

To every candidate who revised the guidelines, memorised the doses,
and still walked out of that room uncertain.

This volume is the bridge between what you know
and what examiners need to see.

HOW TO USE VOLUME TWO

Volume Two builds on the communication, consultation, and core clinical skills developed in Volume One.

This volume focuses on the clinical medicine, specialty, and high-risk presentations commonly encountered in PLAB 2. The emphasis is not on memorising guidelines, but on recognising dangerous conditions, prioritising patient safety, and demonstrating the structured decision-making expected of a UK doctor.

Across ophthalmology, ENT, respiratory medicine, cardiology, diabetes, women's health, paediatrics, psychiatry, surgery, oncology, frailty, safeguarding, and palliative care, the examiner is assessing the same core abilities:

✓ Recognise risk early

✓ Prioritise ABCDE and patient safety

✓ Escalate appropriately

✓ Communicate clearly and professionally

✓ Reassess after intervention

✓ Demonstrate safe NHS practice

Every chapter is structured around examiner expectations and focuses on the actions, verbalisation, and clinical reasoning that generate marks in the examination.

To maximise your score:

1. Read the chapter overview before studying the content.
2. Learn the red flags and escalation triggers.
3. Practise the examiner-facing scripts aloud.
4. Review the Instant Fail sections carefully.
5. Master the Gold Closing Statements.
6. Apply each chapter to mock stations and clinical scenarios.

Remember:

PLAB 2 is not primarily a test of medical knowledge. It is a test of whether you can recognise danger, manage uncertainty, communicate effectively, and keep patients safe.

The candidate who demonstrates safe clinical judgement will consistently outperform the candidate who simply knows the most facts.

AMaC Core Rule:

Recognise Early.
Act Safely.
Escalate Appropriately.
Reassess Frequently.

Think.
Speak.
Perform.

Table of Contents — Volume 2

CLINICAL SYSTEMS & EMERGENCIES

CHAPTER 27 · ACUTE VISION LOSS & EYE EMERGENCIES

CRAO · GCA · Retinal Detachment · Angle Closure · Amaurosis Fugax
EYE-TIME · CHERRY · HEAD-JAW-VIS · FLASH · PAINFUL
CORE · ED/Acute/GP Emergency · CAUTION — HIGH INSTANT FAIL RISK

Abbreviations used in this chapter: **CRAO** Central Retinal Artery Occlusion · **GCA** Giant Cell Arteritis · **RAPD** Relative Afferent Pupillary Defect · **VA** Visual Acuity

THINK — Universal OSCE Identity:
"I am assessing acute vision loss using ABCDE, rapid visual triage (EYE-TIME), immediate identification of sight-threatening pathology, and urgent escalation to prevent irreversible blindness or systemic complications."

Golden Rules:
Visual acuity = GCS of the eye — always first test · Do NOT delay treatment for investigations (especially GCA/CRAO)
Early escalation is mandatory (ophthalmology ± stroke team)

Instant Fail Triggers

✗ Not checking visual acuity FIRST · ✗ Missing RAPD in CRAO / optic nerve disease
✗ Delaying steroids in GCA (blindness risk) · ✗ Treating angle closure as conjunctivitis
✗ Dilating a painful/red eye · ✗ Missing retinal detachment (flashes + curtain)
✗ Not treating CRAO as stroke equivalent · ✗ No urgent ophthalmology referral · ✗ No SBAR escalation

Golden 60-Second Flow

0–10s: Safety + call for help + monitoring
10–30s: ABCDE + visual acuity (FIRST test) + glucose
30–60s: IV access + basic bloods + pattern recognition
🔴 Emergency pathology → treat now | 🟢 Stable → investigate after stabilisation

EYE-TIME Assessment Framework

E	Examine visual acuity FIRST	Use Snellen chart / count fingers / light perception
Y	Why is this emergency?	Time of onset · monocular vs binocular · painful vs painless
E	Examine pupils (RAPD) + fundoscopy	RAPD = afferent defect (optic nerve/retina)
T	Time-critical intervention	Act immediately if CRAO/GCA/angle closure
I	Immediate referral pathway	Ophthalmology ± stroke team

M	Medications if indicated	Steroids/pilocarpine/aspirin
E	Escalate + Explain to patient	SBAR + documentation + safety-net

Condition Overview — Quick Recognition

Condition	Key Features	Mnemonic	Immediate Action
CRAO	Sudden painless monocular loss · cherry red spot · RAPD+	CHERRY	Stroke workup + urgent ophthalmology
GCA	Age >50 · temporal headache · jaw claudication · visual symptoms	HEAD-JAW-VIS	Steroids IMMEDIATELY
Retinal Detachment	Flashes + shower of floaters + curtain over vision	FLASH	Same-day ophthalmology — keep still
Acute Angle Closure	Severe eye pain · mid-dilated fixed pupil · foggy cornea · vomiting	PAINFUL	Pilocarpine + acetazolamide — do NOT dilate
Amaurosis Fugax	Transient monocular loss — full recovery	TIA of eye	Aspirin + TIA pathway

CRAO — Ocular Stroke (CHERRY)

Key Features: Sudden painless monocular vision loss · Cherry red spot on fundoscopy · RAPD positive

Immediate Actions:

✓ Urgent ophthalmology referral · ✓ Stroke workup: ECG, carotid Doppler, echocardiogram

✓ Consider aspirin if appropriate · ✗ Do NOT wait for spontaneous recovery · ✗ Do NOT treat as isolated eye problem

SAY — Examiner Line: "This is an ocular stroke requiring immediate systemic vascular workup."

GCA — Large Vessel Vasculitis (HEAD-JAW-VIS)

Key Features: Age >50 · Temporal headache · Jaw claudication · Visual symptoms
Immediate Actions:

✓ START steroids immediately — do NOT wait for ESR/biopsy

✓ Oral prednisolone 40–60 mg if no visual loss

✓ IV methylprednisolone 500 mg–1 g + same-day ophthalmology if visual symptoms

✓ Temporal artery biopsy within 1 week

✗ Do NOT delay steroids for ESR · ✗ Do NOT wait for biopsy results

SAY — Examiner Line: "GCA until proven otherwise — steroids must be started immediately to prevent irreversible blindness."

Retinal Detachment — FLASH

Key Features: Flashes of light · Shower of floaters · Curtain/shadow over vision
Immediate Actions:

✓ SAME-DAY ophthalmology referral · ✓ Advise patient to keep still

✗ Do NOT dilate pupil · ✗ Do NOT delay referral

SAY — Examiner Line: "This is retinal detachment until proven otherwise — time-sensitive surgical emergency."

Acute Angle Closure — PAINFUL

Key Features: Severe eye pain · Mid-dilated fixed pupil · Foggy cornea · Nausea/vomiting
Immediate Actions:

✓ Pilocarpine drops · ✓ Acetazolamide · ✓ Analgesia + antiemetics · ✓ Urgent ophthalmology referral

✗ Do NOT dilate eye · ✗ Do NOT treat as conjunctivitis

SAY — Examiner Line: "Acute angle closure glaucoma requiring immediate pressure reduction and urgent ophthalmology intervention."

Amaurosis Fugax — TIA of the Eye

Key Features: Brief transient monocular vision loss · Full recovery
Immediate Actions:

✓ Stroke workup: ECG, carotid Doppler, echocardiogram · ✓ Aspirin · ✓ Same-day TIA pathway

✗ Do NOT dismiss as benign

SAY — Examiner Line: "This is a TIA equivalent and carries a high early stroke risk."

Escalation — SBAR

"I am escalating early to ophthalmology and relevant specialty teams due to time-critical risk of permanent vision loss or systemic vascular pathology."

S	Situation	Acute vision loss with suspected [condition]
B	Background	Risk factors: age, AF, HTN, diabetes, myopia
A	Assessment	VA reduced, RAPD ±, fundoscopy findings
R	Recommendation	Urgent ophthalmology ± stroke team review

Examiner Checklist

✓ Visual acuity first · ✓ RAPD assessed · ✓ Fundoscopy described
✓ CRAO identified + stroke workup · ✓ GCA treated immediately with steroids
✓ Retinal detachment referred same day · ✓ Angle closure treated (no dilation)
✓ SBAR escalation done · ✓ Safety-net + explanation given

8-Minute OSCE Timeline

0–1 min	Recognition + VA first
1–2 min	ABCDE + pupil exam
2–3 min	Fundoscopy + pattern recognition
3–4 min	Immediate treatment
4–5 min	Referral decision
5–6 min	Investigations
6–7 min	Escalation + explanation
7–8 min	Reassessment + summary

Final Exam Mantra

VA → RAPD → FUNDOSCOPY → CHERRY / FLASH / PAINFUL → TREAT → REFER → ESCALATE

Gold Closing Statement:
"I performed ABCDE and prioritised visual acuity as the first test. I identified a sight-threatening emergency using EYE-TIME. Immediate management: steroids for GCA, stroke workup for CRAO, pressure-lowering treatment for angle closure, and urgent referral for retinal detachment. Escalated to ophthalmology and relevant teams with continuous reassessment to prevent permanent vision loss."

VA first always GCS of the eye	RAPD positive CRAO / optic nerve	Cherry red spot CRAO — ocular stroke	GCA steroids now do not wait for ESR	IV steroids + ophth GCA with visual loss
FLASH = detachment same-day referral	No dilation angle closure rule	Pilocarpine + acetaz angle closure treatment	Amaurosis fugax TIA of eye — stroke risk	SBAR escalate named team always

TOP 5 EXAMINER Q&A · ACUTE VISION LOSS & EYE EMERGENCIES

Q1. Sudden painless vision loss in one eye. First diagnosis to exclude?	Central retinal artery occlusion or GCA-related ischaemia; both are time-critical. Same-day ophthalmology and GCA screen.

TOP 5 EXAMINER Q&A · ACUTE VISION LOSS & EYE EMERGENCIES	
Q2. Which features point to giant cell arteritis?	Age over 50, temporal headache, scalp tenderness, jaw claudication, raised ESR/CRP; start high-dose steroids immediately.
Q3. Painful red eye with haloes and a fixed mid-dilated pupil?	Acute angle-closure glaucoma: lie flat, analgesia and antiemetic, urgent same-day ophthalmology for pressure-lowering treatment.
Q4. Flashes, floaters and a curtain over the vision?	Retinal detachment until proven otherwise: urgent same-day ophthalmology referral; do not reassure and discharge.
Q5. What must every eye station include?	Visual acuity in each eye separately: it is the vital sign of the eye and a marked step.
CURVEBALL	The patient with sudden vision loss mentions jaw pain on chewing. Treat as GCA: steroids now, bloods after; sight in the other eye is at risk.

CHAPTER 28 · UPPER AIRWAY & STRIDOR

Epiglottitis · Croup · Foreign Body · Angioedema
AIRWAY FIRST · SAD C · UP HEALS · CICV
CRITICAL · 🔴 RED PATH · CAUTION — CRITICAL INSTANT FAIL RISK

Abbreviations used in this chapter: **CICV** Cannot Intubate, Cannot Ventilate

THINK — Universal OSCE Identity:
"I am managing an upper airway obstruction using immediate airway-safe positioning, early escalation to anaesthetics, avoidance of distressing interventions, and structured differential diagnosis using a RED PATH safety-first approach."

Golden Rules:
▸ Airway obstruction is treated before diagnosis · ▸ Distress can precipitate complete airway collapse
▸ Epiglottitis = DO NOT DISTURB · ▸ Anaesthetics call is immediate, not conditional

Instant Fail

No recognition of stridor as airway emergency · Throat examination in suspected epiglottitis
Lying patient flat · Delayed anaesthetics call · Forced oxygen mask causing distress
Blind finger sweep in foreign body · Separation from parent (paediatrics)
Sedation in airway compromise · Missing quiet stridor (late deterioration sign)
Attempting cannulation before airway control

Golden 60-Second Opening Flow

0–10s: Doorway assessment — do NOT approach
10–30s: Identify stridor + keep upright + parent present
30–60s: Call anaesthetics + prepare airway trolley
SAY — Must-Say: "This is stridor indicating upper airway obstruction. I will assess from the doorway, keep the patient upright, avoid distress, and call anaesthetics immediately."

THINK — AIRWAY FIRST Framework

A	Assess from distance	Doorway only — do NOT approach
I	Immediate anaesthetics call	Not conditional — call NOW
R	Recognise RED PATH	Severity assessment
W	Work of breathing	Stridor severity + accessory muscles
A	Avoid throat exam / avoid supine	Epiglottitis — never examine throat
Y	Your role = buy time	UP HEALS while awaiting expert help
F	Family present	Calm = airway protection — keep parent

I	Involve ENT early	Second call after anaesthetics
R	Request difficult airway trolley	Ready before needed
S	SAD C differential	Epiglottitis · Angioedema · Diphtheria · Croup · Bacterial tracheitis (Staph aureus — severe stridor, toxic, age <6y, needs ITU/anaesthetics)
T	Theatre preparation	Prepare for definitive airway

SAY — Must-Say: "I am using AIRWAY FIRST to ensure safe escalation and avoidance of airway-triggering interventions."

ABCDE — Airway-Dominant Structure

	Component	Assess	Script / Action
A.	Airway	Drooling · voice change · stridor	"I will not approach or examine the throat if epiglottitis is suspected."
B.	Breathing	RR · SpO_2 · accessory muscles	"Quiet stridor may indicate deterioration rather than improvement."
C.	Circulation	Pulse only	Avoid distressing BP/cannulation
D.	Disability	Agitation = airway risk	Do NOT sedate — agitation is protective
E.	Exposure	Brief only · vaccination status	Minimal intervention

SAD C — Differential Diagnosis

Condition	Key Features	Immediate Action
Epiglottitis	Drooling · tripod position · toxic appearance · no cough	DO NOT DISTURB + anaesthetics NOW
Angioedema	Tongue/lip swelling · ACE inhibitor · rapid onset	IM adrenaline + airway escalation
Diphtheria	Grey membrane · unvaccinated · bull neck	Senior + airway protection · antitoxin
Croup	Barking cough · viral · usually non-toxic child	Dexamethasone ± nebulised adrenaline
Foreign body	Sudden choking · witnessed episode	Obstruction algorithm — NEVER blind finger sweep

Condition Management — Details

Epiglottitis — Highest Risk:

✓ Upright position only · ✗ Do NOT examine throat · ✗ Do NOT cannulate if distressing
✓ Keep parent present · ✓ Immediate anaesthetics call · ✓ Prepare theatre intubation
CAUTION — Quiet stridor = impending collapse (NOT improvement)

Croup:

Barking cough · usually non-toxic · Management:
✓ Oral dexamethasone · ✓ Nebulised adrenaline if moderate/severe · ✓ Keep calm + upright
CAUTION — Quiet stridor = exhaustion (RED FLAG)

Foreign Body:

Sudden onset choking episode. Algorithm:
Partial obstruction → encourage cough · Complete obstruction → back blows / abdominal thrusts · Failure → CPR pathway
NEVER blind finger sweep.

Angioedema:

Tongue/lip swelling · ACE inhibitor often present · Management:
✓ IM adrenaline if airway risk · ✓ No routine antihistamine/steroid (RCUK 2021) · ✓ Stop ACE inhibitor · ✓ Early anaesthetics call

Buying Time — UP HEALS

U	Upright position	Optimise airway geometry
P	Parent present	Calm child = reduced airway spasm
H	Heliox (if available)	Reduces airway resistance
E	Nebulised adrenaline	Reduces mucosal oedema
A	Avoid distress	Distress → airway spasm → collapse
L	Low stimulation environment	Quiet, calm, dim
S	Steroids (croup/angioedema)	Dexamethasone or hydrocortisone

SAY — Must-Say: "I am using UP HEALS to stabilise while awaiting definitive airway management."

Escalation Pathway — Fixed Order

1	Anaesthetics	Immediate — not conditional
2	ENT	Second call
3	ICU	If deteriorating
4	Theatre	Prepare for definitive airway

Prepare: Difficult airway trolley · Intubation equipment · Surgical airway readiness

CICV — Last Resort Airway

Indication: Cannot intubate + Cannot ventilate
Procedure: Scalpel–bougie–tube technique (surgical cricothyroidotomy)
SAY — Must-Say: "I am prepared for cricothyroidotomy in a CICV scenario as a last-resort life-saving intervention."

SAY — Communication — Examiner Marks Core

"Please stay with your child and keep them upright. Your calm presence is helping maintain their airway. We are treating this as an airway emergency and senior help is arriving immediately."

Deterioration Signs — Red Flags

Quiet stridor · Reduced agitation (fatigue) · Falling SpO_2 · Cyanosis · Silent chest
Reduced work of breathing = EXHAUSTION, NOT IMPROVEMENT
SAY — "Less noise does not mean improvement — it may indicate airway failure."

Examiner Checklist

✓ Stridor recognised as airway emergency · ✓ Doorway assessment performed · ✓ AIRWAY FIRST verbalised

✓ Immediate anaesthetics call made · ✓ No throat exam in epiglottitis · ✓ Upright positioning

✓ Parent kept with child · ✓ SAD C used correctly · ✓ UP HEALS applied

✓ Correct foreign body algorithm · ✓ Correct angioedema treatment · ✓ CICV awareness stated

✓ Deterioration signs identified

Final Exam Mantra

Stridor = RED PATH → Doorway → Anaesthetics → No throat exam → Upright → SAD C → UP HEALS → Prepare airway failure

Gold Closing Statement:
"This is upper airway obstruction until proven otherwise. I assessed from the doorway, maintained airway-safe positioning, avoided distressing interventions, escalated immediately to anaesthetics, applied the SAD C differential, initiated UP HEALS for stabilisation, and prepared for definitive airway management including ENT involvement and potential surgical airway if required."

Stridor = red path immediate response	Doorway assess never approach first	Anaesthetics NOW not conditional	No throat exam epiglottitis rule	Upright always never lay flat
Parent with child calm = airway	Quiet stridor worse not better	SAD C differential structured approach	UP HEALS buy time safely	CICV ready last resort airway

TOP 5 EXAMINER Q&A · UPPER AIRWAY & STRIDOR	
Q1. What does stridor at rest tell you?	Significant upper airway obstruction: do not distress the patient, give oxygen, and call anaesthetics and ENT immediately.
Q2. Suspected epiglottitis. What must you avoid?	Examining the throat or lying the patient flat; keep them calm and upright with senior airway help on the way.
Q3. How do you treat moderate croup?	Single dose of oral dexamethasone; nebulised adrenaline with senior input if severe.
Q4. Complete choking obstruction in an adult?	5 back blows, then 5 abdominal thrusts, alternating; CPR if they become unconscious.
Q5. Anaphylaxis vs other causes of stridor?	Look for rapid onset, urticaria, lip and tongue swelling, and a trigger: adrenaline 0.5 mg IM without delay.
CURVEBALL	A child with suspected epiglottitis cries when you approach with a tongue depressor. Stop: examination can precipitate complete obstruction; await senior airway support.

CHAPTER 29 · ACUTE UROLOGICAL & SCROTAL EMERGENCIES

Torsion · Retention · Fournier's · Urosepsis · Paraphimosis

CORE · Surgical Acute Take · CAUTION — INSTANT FAIL RISK

Abbreviations used in this chapter: **AKI** Acute Kidney Injury · **LMWH** Low Molecular Weight Heparin · **VTE** Venous Thromboembolism

THINK — Universal OSCE Identity:
"I manage time-critical urological emergencies using ABCDE, rapid recognition of life-threatening pathology, immediate escalation, and safe stabilisation – avoiding harmful delays."
Examiner Focus: Speed of recognition · Early escalation (before full diagnosis) · Avoidance of dangerous actions · Safety-first decisions

Master Spine — IDENTIFY → ACT → ESCALATE

IDENTIFY → RED / STABLE → ACT (1–2 min) → ESCALATE → REASSESS

Path	Condition	Action
RED	Torsion · Fournier's · Urosepsis+obstruction · Paraphimosis (failed reduction) · Retention+sepsis/AKI	Act NOW + Escalate
STABLE	Epididymo-orchitis · mild infection · painless chronic retention	Investigate then treat

Instant Fail Triggers (NEVER / ALWAYS)

✗ NEVER	✓ ALWAYS
Wait for ultrasound in torsion	Call urology within 2 minutes
Catheterise with blood at meatus / pelvic fracture	Stop – NO catheter
Miss absent cremasteric reflex	Check both sides
Delay antibiotics in sepsis	Sepsis Six within 1 hour
Miss Fournier's extension	Examine perineum + perianal + buttocks + inner thighs
Discharge suspected torsion	Escalate + admit

Golden 60-Second Flow

Time	Action
0–10s	ABCDE + identify emergency (sudden pain? vomiting?)
10–20s	RED flags: absent cremasteric? high-riding testis?

Time	Action
20–30s	TWIST score (≥5 = theatre; 3–4 = urology + US only if no delay)
30–45s	CALL urology (torsion/Fournier's) OR SEPSIS SIX (urosepsis)
45–60s	Manual detorsion / paraphimosis reduction / safe catheter

Testicular Torsion — Time is Testis

TWIST score ≥5 → theatre immediately — no imaging delay.
TWIST 3–4 → urology + ultrasound only if no delay to surgical review.
Manual Detorsion:
Left testis → rotate clockwise (from patient's view) · Right testis → rotate counter-clockwise
180–360 degrees. If pain increases → reverse direction.
Consent: "Bilateral orchidopexy – contralateral testis fixed (bell-clapper is bilateral in 40–50%)."
CAUTION — TRAP: Previous orchidopexy does NOT exclude torsion.

Fournier's Gangrene — Surgical Emergency

FOUR D's: Discolouration · Deep pain (out of proportion) · Debris/crepitus · Deterioration
Examine: perineum + perianal + buttocks + inner thighs — all areas.
Action:
✓ Immediate surgical referral (urology + general surgery) · ✓ IV antibiotics + fluids
✓ LRINEC score (≥6 high risk — but normal does NOT exclude) · ✓ Check blood glucose (40–60% diabetic)

Urosepsis — Sepsis Six + Source Control

Sepsis Six (within 1 hour):
Oxygen → Blood cultures → IV antibiotics → IV fluids → Lactate → Urine output
Source Control = RELIEVE OBSTRUCTION: Catheter / stent / nephrostomy OR drain abscess
Add: VTE assessment + prophylactic LMWH (sepsis = pro-thrombotic)

Paraphimosis — Reduce Before Calling

Analgesia first: Dorsal nerve block (2% lignocaine no adrenaline)

Step	Technique	Notes
1	Ice	Reduces oedema
2	Compression	Wrap/squeeze glans to reduce swelling
3	Osmotic reduction	Sugar or glucose gauze over glans
4	Manual reduction	Push glans through foreskin
5	Dundee technique	Multiple needle punctures to release oedema

Step	Technique	Notes
6	Failed → urology	Dorsal slit or circumcision

Acute Urinary Retention — RED if Sepsis/AKI

Safe Catheterisation — 5 Cs:
Check urethral injury · Correct size · Clean aseptic · Cuff with sterile water ONLY · Collect urine
High PVR >800 mL: Consider catheter valve or intermittent catheterisation
Post-obstructive diuresis: Monitor BP/electrolytes — do NOT clamp (not evidence-based)
✗ NEVER catheterise with blood at meatus or suspected pelvic fracture.

Green Path — Stable Conditions

Condition	Action
Epididymo-orchitis	Urinalysis + MSU + STI screen (<35) + antibiotics (cover STI or UTI)
Painless chronic retention	Elective catheterisation or trial without catheter
Mild infection	Outpatient care

SAY — Escalation Line — Say Exactly

"I am escalating immediately to [urology/general surgery] due to a time-critical emergency. This is [torsion/Fournier's/sepsis/paraphimosis]. I have [immediate action]. I will reassess."

Examiner Checklist

✓ Time documented · ✓ Torsion recognised early + TWIST score
✓ Urology called immediately — no imaging delay · ✓ Manual detorsion attempted
✓ Urethral injury excluded — safe catheterisation · ✓ Sepsis Six + source control
✓ Fournier's full perineal examination · ✓ Paraphimosis reduced or escalated
✓ Escalation verbalised · ✓ Reassessment stated

Final Exam Mantra

Torsion → call before palpating.
Fournier's → examine before referring.
Urosepsis → antibiotics before cultures.
Paraphimosis → reduce before calling.
Retention → check urethra first.

Gold Closing Statement:

"I identified a time-critical urological emergency. I escalated immediately – torsion called urology within 2 minutes without imaging. Fournier's – full perineal exam + surgical referral. Urosepsis – Sepsis Six with source control. Paraphimosis – reduction with analgesia. I will reassess after every intervention."

Torsion call urology before imaging	TWIST ≥5 theatre immediately	Bell-clapper bilateral orchidopexy	Fournier's examine perineum fully	FOUR D's Discolouration · Deep pain · Debris · Deterioration
Urosepsis Sepsis Six + source control	No catheter blood at meatus rule	Paraphimosis reduce before calling	5 Cs catheter safe catheterisation	Post-obstructive monitor, do not clamp

TOP 5 EXAMINER Q&A · ACUTE UROLOGICAL & SCROTAL EMERGENCIES	
Q1. Acute scrotal pain in a teenager. Default diagnosis?	Testicular torsion until proven otherwise: urgent urology referral; the window is roughly 6 hours.
Q2. Does a normal cremasteric reflex exclude torsion?	No clinical sign reliably excludes it; if suspected, refer for surgical exploration rather than waiting for imaging.
Q3. How do you manage acute urinary retention?	Catheterise, record the residual volume, treat the cause, and check renal function.
Q4. What is Fournier's gangrene and the key action?	Necrotising infection of the perineum: IV antibiotics and immediate surgical debridement; senior escalation at once.
Q5. Infected, obstructed kidney. Why is it an emergency?	Pus under pressure destroys the kidney and drives sepsis: urgent decompression by nephrostomy or stent.
CURVEBALL	Ultrasound is available in two hours for suspected torsion. Do not wait: this is a clinical diagnosis and delayed exploration loses the testis.

CHAPTER 30 · CARDIOVASCULAR RISK & DIABETES ANNUAL REVIEW

6-PACK · TARGET · LOOK-FEEL · M-S-G-I · DRIVE-5 · SADMAN

HbA1c Individualisation · QRISK3 · Foot Examination · SGLT2i/GLP-1 · Insulin Safety · Shared Decision-Making

CRITICAL · CORE STATION · CAUTION — HIGH INSTANT FAIL RISK

Abbreviations used in this chapter: **AKI** Acute Kidney Injury · **DKA** Diabetic Ketoacidosis · **DVLA** Driver & Vehicle Licensing Agency · **GLP-1** Glucagon-Like Peptide-1 agonist · **QRISK3** QRISK3 cardiovascular risk score · **SGLT2** Sodium-Glucose Cotransporter-2 inhibitor

Core Exam Focus:
Complication screening · Cardiovascular risk management · Medication safety and escalation · Lifestyle and social tailoring · Shared decision-making

Examiner Lens: "Can this candidate deliver safe, structured, patient-centred long-term diabetes care?"

Marks come from: Verbal structure · Prioritisation · Safety-netting · Communication clarity · Clinical completeness

Instant Fail Triggers:
Same HbA1c target for all patients · No foot examination · Missing Charcot foot
No insulin driving advice · Unsafe sick day advice · Poor cardiovascular risk explanation
No social tailoring · No shared decision-making · No safety netting

THINK — Core Rule: Diabetes annual review = complications + cardiovascular risk + safety + individualisation.

Golden Opening Script

"Welcome to your diabetes annual review. Today I'd like to review your blood sugar control, cardiovascular risk, medications, and check for complications affecting your eyes, kidneys, and feet. We'll also discuss safety issues like hypos, driving, and sick day rules, and agree a plan together."

"Are there any particular concerns you'd like us to focus on today?"

"Before we begin, could you talk me through your current diabetes medications and how you are taking them?"

6-PACK Framework

P	Prioritise Targets (HbA1c)	Individualise using TARGET
A	Assess Complications	Eyes · Kidneys · Feet
C	Cardiovascular Risk	QRISK3 · BP · Cholesterol · Smoking
K	Knowledge & Safety	Hypoglycaemia · Sick day rules · Driving
E	Escalate Treatment	M-S-G-I pathway

T	Tailor Care	Occupation · Cost · Literacy · Culture · Fasting · Disability

HbA1c Individualisation — TARGET

T	Treatment burden	Complexity of current regimen
A	Age	Older patients → more relaxed targets
R	Risk of hypoglycaemia	Driver, lives alone, impaired awareness
G	General frailty	Frail → relaxed target
E	Existing complications	Established CVD → individualise
T	Time to benefit	Limited life expectancy → relaxed target

Exam Anchor: "For many adults, NICE often uses HbA1c targets around 48 mmol/mol, but targets must always be individualised using TARGET."
SAY — Script: "Your HbA1c is [X], and the trend is [improving/stable/worsening]. Using TARGET, I would individualise your goal based on your overall health and risk of hypoglycaemia. What feels realistic for you?"

Cardiovascular Risk — QRISK3

"Your QRISK3 score estimates your risk of heart attack or stroke over the next 10 years."

100-Person Explanation: "A risk of [X]% means that out of 100 people similar to you, about [X] may have a heart attack or stroke in the next 10 years."

Statin Discussion: "Statins significantly reduce cardiovascular risk. The decision is shared and based on what matters to you."

Blood Pressure: "Your BP is [X]. Controlling blood pressure protects your heart, brain, kidneys, and eyes."

Foot Examination — LOOK-FEEL

L	LOOK: Inspect	Toes · Soles · Heels · Pressure areas
O	Observe footwear	"Let's check your footwear — poorly fitting shoes commonly cause ulcers."
O	One-minute monofilament	Loss of sensation = neuropathy risk
K	Key pulses	Dorsalis pedis · Posterior tibial
F	Feel temperature	Warm = infection/Charcot · Cold = vascular disease
E	Evaluate risk	Low · Increased · High
E	Educate	Self-care + footwear + warning signs

Charcot Foot — Emergency:
Red · Hot · Swollen · Painless
"This is suspicious for Charcot foot, which is an emergency. Do not weight-bear. I am arranging urgent specialist foot team review today."

Medication Escalation — M-S-G-I

	Drug	Key Script
M	Metformin	First-line — check eGFR/tolerability
S	SGLT2 inhibitor	"This medication protects the heart and kidneys beyond glucose control."
G	GLP-1 receptor agonist	"Helps with blood sugar and weight. Nausea common initially. Some are once-weekly injections."
I	Insulin	Check driving before starting. NEVER stop during illness — dose adjust instead.

Driving Rules — DRIVE-5

SAY — Ask first: "Do you drive?"

1	Test BG ≥5.0 mmol/L before EVERY journey. Do NOT drive if BG <5.0 mmol/L. Check every 2 hours on long journeys. Always carry rapid-acting glucose in the vehicle. NOTIFY DVLA if insulin-treated (mandatory).	Every time
2	Recheck every 2 hours	Long journeys
3	Hypo while driving → STOP immediately	Pull over safely
4	Hypo while driving: STOP safely, remove keys, move to passenger seat. Treat hypo. Wait 45 MINUTES minimum before driving again (not just until BG normalises). Document episode.	Not 15 — 45 minutes
5	Carry glucose in vehicle at all times	Mandatory

Hypoglycaemia Treatment — FAST 15-20:
15–20g fast-acting carbohydrate (glucose tablets, juice) · Recheck BM in 15 minutes

Sick Day Rules — SADMAN

	Drug	Action During Illness
S	SGLT2 inhibitor	STOP — risk of DKA during illness (including euglycaemic DKA — glucose may be only mildly elevated; do not rely on glucose alone to exclude DKA when on SGLT2 inhibitor)
A	ACEi/ARBs	STOP — AKI risk
D	Diuretics	STOP — dehydration risk
M	Metformin	STOP — lactic acidosis risk

	Drug	Action During Illness
A	Monitor	Check glucose more often during illness
N	NSAIDs	STOP — AKI risk

Insulin Safety Addition:
"If you take insulin, do NOT stop it completely during illness. You may need dose adjustment, but stopping insulin entirely can cause dangerous hyperglycaemia or diabetic ketoacidosis."

Social & Cultural Care

Ask about: Smoking · Occupation · Cost · Interpreter · Literacy · Fasting (Ramadan)
"Smoking significantly increases cardiovascular risk. Would you like support to stop?"
"Healthy eating does not need to be expensive — we can adapt advice to your situation."
"Are you planning to fast for Ramadan? We can adjust your medication safely."

Complications Screening · Vaccinations

Eyes: "When was your last diabetic retinal screening? Usually annual. If overdue, I will refer you."
Kidneys: "I'd review eGFR and urine albumin-to-creatinine ratio (ACR) to detect early kidney disease and guide medication choice."
Vaccinations: "Annual flu vaccination and appropriate pneumococcal vaccination recommended."
Teach-back: "Just to check I've explained clearly — could you tell me what you would do if you had a hypo?"

Follow-Up & Safety Netting

Situation	Follow-Up Interval
Stable, well-controlled	Annual review
Medication change	3 months
Poor control	3–6 months
High-risk feet	More frequent podiatry
New insulin	Early review

Safety Netting — Return if:
Recurrent hypos · Foot redness/swelling · Vomiting or dehydration · DKA symptoms · Unexpected weight loss

Instant Fail Behaviours

No HbA1c individualisation · No foot exam · Missed Charcot foot
Unsafe insulin advice · No driving assessment · Poor QRISK explanation
No social tailoring · No safety netting

Final Exam Mantra

6-PACK → TARGET HbA1c → QRISK3 → LOOK-FEEL feet → M-S-G-I escalation → DRIVE-5 → SADMAN → Social tailoring → Teach-back → Safety-net

Gold Closing Statement:

"To summarise, your HbA1c is [X] and we have individualised your target using TARGET. Your cardiovascular risk has been discussed using QRISK3, and we have reviewed your medications, kidney function, and foot health. We have also covered safety issues including hypoglycaemia, driving rules, and sick day guidance. Our plan is [X], with follow-up in [Y]. Please seek help earlier if any red flag symptoms develop. Do you have any questions?"

6-PACK framework structured annual review	TARGET HbA1c never one-size-fits-all	LOOK-FEEL feet every annual review	Charcot = emergency no weight-bearing	M-S-G-I escalation stepwise treatment
DRIVE-5 insulin + driving rules	SADMAN sick day stop these 4 drugs	Insulin never stop dose adjust, not stop	QRISK3 + statins shared decision	Safety-net always red flags + follow-up

TOP 5 EXAMINER Q&A · CARDIOVASCULAR RISK & DIABETES ANNUAL REVIEW

Q1. What does QRISK3 estimate and what follows a score of 10% or more?	Ten-year cardiovascular risk; discuss and offer atorvastatin 20 mg alongside lifestyle change, as a shared decision.
Q2. How do you individualise an HbA1c target?	Balance age, frailty, hypoglycaemia risk and comorbidity: roughly 48 for the young and fit, relaxed to 53 or higher in frailty.
Q3. What does the diabetic foot check include?	Inspection, foot pulses and 10 g monofilament sensation, with risk stratification and podiatry referral as indicated.
Q4. Which annual screens does a diabetic review include?	Retinal screening, urine ACR and renal function, feet, blood pressure, lipids and HbA1c.
Q5. The patient declines a statin. What do you do?	Explore concerns, give absolute-risk information, respect the decision, document it, and keep the door open for review.
CURVEBALL	The patient asks "will I be on these tablets forever?" Explain honestly: treatment is long-term while risk persists, but always reviewable: this is a partnership, not a sentence.

CHAPTER 31 · RESPIRATORY REVIEWS

Asthma & COPD Annual Management

SALT · PRESSED · SMILE · BREATHE · MART · GOLD · Three As · Ask–Advise–Act

CORE · GP / Respiratory Clinic · CAUTION — HIGH INSTANT FAIL RISK

Abbreviations used in this chapter: **COPD** Chronic Obstructive Pulmonary Disease · **DPI** Dry Powder Inhaler · **DVLA** Driver & Vehicle Licensing Agency · **LABA** Long-Acting Beta-Agonist · **MART** Maintenance & Reliever Therapy · **MRC** Medical Research Council scale · **SABA** Short-Acting Beta-Agonist

Core Exam Idea: Respiratory review = Control + Technique + Adherence + Safety + Stepwise escalation

Examiner Lens: "Can this candidate optimise inhalers safely, prevent exacerbations, and recognise deterioration early?"

Marks come from: Inhaler technique · Recognising poor control · Safe escalation · Smoking intervention · Patient education · Action planning · Safety-netting

THINK — Core Rule: Most uncontrolled asthma/COPD is caused by poor technique, poor adherence, or smoking — not lack of medication.

Instant Fail Triggers:

No inhaler technique check · Assume adherence is good · Step up without Three As

Forget rinse & spit after ICS · Miss pMDI vs DPI distinction · No smoking discussion

No action plan · Unsafe MART explanation · No safety-netting

Golden Opening Script

"Thank you for coming in today. I'd like to review your breathing symptoms, check how well your inhalers are working and being used, and see whether any treatment changes are needed to help prevent flare-ups and keep you well."

"I'll also ask about smoking, triggers, and safety issues. Is that okay?"

8-Minute Review Flow

0–1 min	Introduction + purpose
1–2 min	Assess symptom control
2–3 min	Inhaler technique check (MAJOR MARK AREA)
3–4 min	Adherence + smoking + triggers
4–5 min	Three As before escalation
5–6 min	Stepwise management
6–7 min	Education + action plan
7–8 min	Safety-net + follow-up

1 Assess Control

Ask About	Red Flags
Daytime symptoms	Increasing reliever use
Night waking	Night symptoms
Reliever use frequency	Recent hospital admission
Exercise limitation	Frequent oral steroids
Exacerbations + admissions	Worsening exercise tolerance

Controlled Asthma Anchor: Reliever ≤2/week · No night symptoms · Minimal activity limitation
SAY — Must-Say: "Frequent flare-ups or increased reliever use suggest poor control and mean we should review treatment and inhaler use carefully."

2 Inhaler Technique — PRESSED (pMDI) vs DPI

Golden Rule: Never assume inhaler technique is correct.
SAY — Always say: "Please show me how you use your inhaler."

	PRESSED (pMDI)	DPI	Common Errors
P	Prepare: shake + remove cap	Load dose (twist/click)	Not shaking pMDI
R	Respire out gently	Breathe out gently	Breathing out into mouthpiece
E	Engage: seal lips	Seal lips	Poor lip seal
S	Squeeze: press at start of inhale	N/A — no actuation	Pressing before inhaling
S	Slow deep breath in	QUICK deep breath in	pMDI too fast · DPI too slow
E	Expire: hold breath 5–10s	Hold breath 5–10s	Not holding breath
D	Do again: wait 30–60s	Wait before repeat	Multiple puffs together

ICS Safety — Automatic Mark Phrase: "After using your steroid inhaler, rinse your mouth and spit out the water to prevent oral thrush."

3 Spacer Education — SMILE

When to Use: pMDI users · Poor coordination · Recurrent exacerbations · High-dose ICS

S	Shake + insert	Shake inhaler and insert into spacer
M	Make seal	Seal lips around spacer mouthpiece

I	Inhale slowly	One puff → breathe in slowly
L	Listen	Whistle = breathing in too fast
E	Exhale away	Breathe out away from mouthpiece

Cleaning: Wash weekly in warm soapy water · Air dry naturally · Do NOT towel dry

4 Three As — Before Any Step-Up

Must-Say Safety Rule: Before increasing treatment, always check Three As first.

A	Adherence	"Are you taking it regularly?"
A	Assessment of technique	"Can you show me how you use it?"
A	Alternative diagnosis	"Could another diagnosis or trigger be contributing?"

5 Asthma Management — SALT

	SALT	Detail
S	SABA only	Rare — only if symptoms are infrequent
A	ADD ICS	Low-dose inhaled corticosteroid
L	ADD LABA	Combination ICS/LABA inhaler
T	THINK MART	One inhaler as BOTH preventer and reliever

MART Safety Scripts:

"Your combination inhaler is now your main preventer and reliever inhaler. You usually no longer need routine blue inhaler use."

"Keep your blue inhaler as a backup in case your MART inhaler is unavailable."

Step-Down Rule: Only consider stepping down if stable ≥3 months. Reduce gradually. Do NOT stop ICS abruptly.

6 Action Plan — Green / Amber / Red

Zone	Status	Action
GREEN	Well controlled	Continue usual treatment
AMBER	Worsening symptoms	Increase treatment as advised
RED	Severe symptoms / poor response	Seek urgent medical help

Must-Say Safety-Net: "Please seek urgent help if your inhaler is not relieving symptoms, you are struggling to speak, or your breathing rapidly worsens."

7 COPD Review — BREATHE + GOLD Staging

Confirm Diagnosis: "COPD is confirmed by post-bronchodilator spirometry showing FEV1/FVC below 0.7."

GOLD Stage	FEV1 %	Severity
GOLD 1	≥80%	Mild
GOLD 2	50–79%	Moderate
GOLD 3	30–49%	Severe
GOLD 4	<30%	Very severe

	BREATHE	Detail
B	Bronchodilators	SABA/SAMA → LABA/LAMA → combination
R	Review symptoms + exacerbations	Frequent exacerbations → escalate
E	Escalate treatment	ICS only if ≥2 exacerbations/year
A	Action plan	Written plan for worsening
T	Treat comorbidities	AF, heart failure, depression, osteoporosis
H	Healthy lifestyle + pulmonary rehab	MRC grade 3–5 → refer
E	Every review check technique	Always — no exceptions

Rescue Packs: ≥2 exacerbations/year → consider pre-supplied steroids + antibiotics with clear instructions.
Pulmonary Rehab: "Pulmonary rehabilitation can improve breathlessness, exercise tolerance, and reduce hospital admissions."

8 Smoking · Preventative Care · DVLA · Follow-Up

Ask–Advise–Act:
Ask: "Do you currently smoke or vape?"
Advise: "Stopping smoking is the single most effective thing you can do for your lungs."
Act: Offer nicotine replacement · Stop smoking referral · Medication support
Vaping Script: "Vaping is less harmful than smoking and may help some people quit, but the goal is to become nicotine-free."

Follow-Up	Interval
Stable	Annual review
Treatment changed	4–6 weeks
Poor control	Earlier review

Preventative Care: Annual flu vaccination · Pneumococcal vaccination · Smoking cessation support
DVLA: Consider if disabling symptoms / severe breathlessness / long-term oxygen therapy
Occupational trigger: "Do your symptoms improve when away from work?"

Examiner Checklist

✓ Control assessed · ✓ Inhaler demonstrated by patient · ✓ pMDI vs DPI corrected
✓ Rinse & spit advised · ✓ Adherence checked · ✓ Smoking addressed
✓ Occupational trigger asked · ✓ Three As completed · ✓ SALT applied correctly
✓ MART explained safely · ✓ COPD confirmed with spirometry · ✓ GOLD stage recognised
✓ Pulmonary rehab offered · ✓ Action plan given · ✓ Safety-netting provided

Final Exam Mantra

CONTROL → TECHNIQUE → ADHERENCE → THREE As → STEP-UP → ACTION PLAN → SAFETY NET
pMDI = slow · DPI = quick · ICS = rinse & spit · MART = main reliever · COPD = FEV1/FVC <0.7
Treat the inhaler before escalating the inhaler.

Gold Closing Summary:
"Today we reviewed your respiratory symptoms, inhaler technique, and current treatment. Your control is currently [controlled/partially/uncontrolled]. I've checked your inhaler technique and discussed ways to improve symptom control and reduce flare-ups. We've reviewed smoking and triggers, agreed a treatment plan, and discussed what to do if symptoms worsen. Please come back sooner if you need your reliever more often, develop worsening breathlessness, or your inhalers stop helping."

Show me technique always, never assume	pMDI = slow inhale DPI = quick inhale	Rinse & spit ICS auto-mark phrase	Three As first before any step-up	SALT framework asthma escalation
MART = main reliever explain clearly	COPD FEV1/FVC <0.7 spirometry diagnosis	GOLD staging 1–4 by FEV1%	Pulmonary rehab MRC grade 3–5	Safety-net always inhaler stopping helping

TOP 5 EXAMINER Q&A · RESPIRATORY REVIEWS	
Q1. What defines poor asthma control at review?	Three or more days a week with symptoms or reliever use, night waking, or any recent attack; check technique and adherence first.
Q2. What is MART?	Maintenance and reliever therapy: one combined ICS/formoterol inhaler used regularly and as required.
Q3. What must you check before stepping up treatment?	Inhaler technique, adherence, triggers and smoking: most "treatment failure" is technique failure.
Q4. Key components of a COPD review?	Symptom burden (CAT/MRC), exacerbation count, inhaler technique, smoking cessation, vaccination, and pulmonary rehabilitation.
Q5. When do you suspect something beyond COPD?	Haemoptysis, weight loss, disproportionate breathlessness or chest pain: investigate, do not label.

TOP 5 EXAMINER Q&A · RESPIRATORY REVIEWS	
CURVEBALL	The patient's technique is perfect but control is poor, and they smoke. Smoking cessation is the single most effective intervention: address it before escalating drugs.

CHAPTER 32 · WOMEN'S HEALTH I

Contraception & Sexual Health

SAFER SEX · 5Ps · UKMEC · LARC-UPS · CUP FIRST · TRACE · OPEN · FORCED · FRAZER

CRITICAL CORE · CAUTION — HIGH INSTANT FAIL RISK

Abbreviations used in this chapter: **COC** Combined Oral Contraceptive · **HPV** Human Papillomavirus · **IUD** Intrauterine Device · **IUS** Intrauterine System · **LARC** Long-Acting Reversible Contraception · **LNG** Levonorgestrel · **LNG-IUS** Levonorgestrel Intrauterine System · **PID** Pelvic Inflammatory Disease · **POP** Progestogen-Only Pill · **UKMEC** UK Medical Eligibility Criteria · **UPA** Ulipristal Acetate · **UPSI** Unprotected Sexual Intercourse · **VTE** Venous Thromboembolism

Examiner Lens: "Will this doctor provide safe, inclusive, evidence-based care while knowing when to escalate?"

Examiner checks: Safety (UKMEC + ectopic) · Structure · Inclusive communication · STI/TRACE · Escalation recognition

SAY — Golden Minute Opening:

"Thank you for coming in. Everything we discuss is confidential. I'll use the SAFER SEX framework — screening for pregnancy and safeguarding, checking medical safety, discussing contraception options, offering STI testing, and making a plan together. Some questions are personal — is that OK?"

Instant Fail Triggers

No sexual history · UKMEC 4 missed · Oestrogen prescribed when unsafe
Wrong EC hierarchy · Copper IUD not offered for EC · Missed ectopic pregnancy
No STI testing offered · No safeguarding assessment · HIV PEP offered after 72h
No FRAZER in under-16s · No red flag escalation · No safety-netting

SAFER SEX — Chapter Spine

	Meaning	What to Cover
S	Screening	Pregnancy risk + safeguarding (5Ps + FORCED)
A	Assess UKMEC	Contraindications — AURA = 4
F	Failure rates	LARC >99% effective
E	Emergency contraception	CUP FIRST: Cu-IUD > UPA > LNG
R	Regular contraception	LARC-UPS framework
S	STI testing	TRACE + vaccination
E	Equality	OPEN inclusive care
X	HIV prevention	PEP + PrEP

8-Minute OSCE Map (3–3–1–1):
0–3 min: History: 5Ps + FORCED + red flags
3–6 min: Discussion: UKMEC + contraception options
6–7 min: STI/HIV: Testing + TRACE + PEP/PrEP
7–8 min: Closing: Safety-net + follow-up + teach-back

5Ps-UK Sexual History

SAY — Framing: "I ask everyone these questions because it helps me give safe advice."

Topic	Questions
Partners	New partners? Male, female, or both?
Practices	Vaginal, anal, oral?
Protection	Condoms? Previous contraception?
Pregnancy plans	Trying to conceive now or later?
Past STIs	Previous infections or treatment?
UKMEC risks	Aura, smoking, VTE, BMI, liver disease

CAUTION — UKMEC Safety — AURA = 4

Migraine with aura = UKMEC 4 = NO combined pill.

Category	Conditions
UKMEC 4 — NO	Migraine with aura · Current breast cancer · Active liver disease · Smoker ≥35 + ≥15 cigarettes/day
UKMEC 3 — CAUTION	Smoker ≥35 + <15/day · BMI >35 · Controlled hypertension
VTE counselling	"Clot risk on combined pill is ~5–12 per 10,000/year — lower than during pregnancy."

Contraception — LARC-UPS

SAY — LARC First: "Long-acting methods are over 99% effective — fit and forget."

	LARC-UPS	Detail
L	LARC first	Copper IUD (5–10yr) · LNG-IUS (5–8yr) · Implant (3yr)
A	Ask preferences	Bleeding patterns · Hormones · Convenience
R	Recommend suitable options	Based on UKMEC + preferences
C	Check UKMEC safety	Mandatory before prescribing

	LARC-UPS	Detail
U	User-dependent if LARC declined	COC · POP · Depo-Provera
P	Provide counselling	Acne→COC · Heavy periods→LNG-IUS · Breastfeeding→POP/IUS/implant
S	Summarise + confirm decision	Shared decision-making

Emergency Contraception — CUP FIRST

Hierarchy: Copper IUD > Ulipristal (UPA) > Levonorgestrel (LNG)

Method	Window	Key Points
Copper IUD	Up to 5 days	Most effective (>99%) · Not affected by weight · Enzyme inducers: preferred
Ulipristal (UPA)	Up to 5 days	More effective than LNG closer to ovulation · BMI >35 or >80kg: IUD preferred
Levonorgestrel (LNG)	Best <72h	Can start hormonal contraception immediately after · BMI >30 or >70kg: IUD preferred

After EC — Starting Contraception:
After LNG: Start immediately · After UPA: Delay 5 days · After Copper IUD: Already effective
Vomiting within 3h: Repeat dose or offer IUD · Breastfeeding: Prefer LNG

Missed Pill Rules

Scenario	Action
COC <48h late	Take and continue pack
COC ≥48h or 3+ missed	Take last missed · Continue pack · Condoms 7 days · If week 1 + UPSI → consider EC
Traditional POP >3h late	Condoms for 2 days · If first 7 days + UPSI in previous 7 days → EC
Desogestrel POP >12h late	Condoms for 2 days

Depo-Provera (DMPA): Every 12–13 weeks · Review bone health after 2 years · Fertility return may take up to 1 year

STI Testing + TRACE Partner Notification

	TRACE	Meaning
T	Tell partners	Inform recent contacts

	TRACE	Meaning
R	Refer to health advisor	Specialist support available
A	Anonymous notification available	Without patient disclosing name
C	Condoms until treated	Both partners
E	Ensure follow-up	Test of cure where needed

Full STI Screen: Chlamydia/Gonorrhoea (urine or swab) · HIV/Syphilis (blood) · Hep B/C if risk · Herpes (lesion swab)
Vaccination: HPV catch-up up to age 25 · Hep B for MSM, sex workers, PWID

HIV Prevention — PEP & PrEP

PEP Key Rule: Must start within 72 hours — ideally within 24h.
28-day course · Baseline HIV test + 4 weeks + 12 weeks
"PEP is started after baseline HIV testing, but treatment should not be delayed if risk is high."
"Do NOT use PrEP for post-exposure treatment."

PrEP: Daily (one tablet) OR event-based (MSM only)
Monitoring: HIV test before starting · Renal function · STI screening every 3 months
CAUTION — Do not start if symptoms suggest acute HIV · "PrEP does not protect against pregnancy or other STIs."

Inclusive Practice · OPEN · FORCED · FRAZER

	OPEN (Inclusive)	FORCED (Safeguarding)
O/F	Open questions	Forced sex/coercion
P/O	Pronouns: ask preferred pronouns	Older partner
E/R	Explore anatomy without assumptions	Repeated STIs
N/C	Neutral language throughout	Controlling behaviour
-/E	-	Exploitation
-/D	-	Distress/fear

FRAZER — Under-16 Confidentiality:

F — Fully understands · R — Refuses parental involvement · A — At risk without treatment

Z — Will continue sexual activity regardless · E — Encourage parental involvement · R — Record clearly

CAUTION — Significant age gap may require safeguarding referral.

Escalation — Stop and Act Now

STOP contraception discussion and escalate immediately if:

CAUTION — Suspected ectopic pregnancy · CAUTION — PID with sepsis · CAUTION — Acute HIV seroconversion · CAUTION — Safeguarding emergency

Ectopic Red Flags: CAUTION — Positive pregnancy test + pain or bleeding · CAUTION — One-sided pain · CAUTION — Shoulder-tip pain · CAUTION — Collapse/syncope

"Any positive pregnancy test with pain or bleeding is ectopic until proven otherwise."

Follow-Up & Safety Netting

Situation	Follow-up
New contraception	3 months
IUD/IUS/Implant	4–6 weeks
PEP	Day 3–5, week 4, week 12
PrEP	Every 3 months

Return Urgently If: Severe pelvic pain · Heavy bleeding · Fever/discharge · Positive test after EC · Cannot feel implant · Severe post-IUD pain

Examiner Checklist

✓ Confidentiality established · ✓ Sexual history completed · ✓ UKMEC assessed

✓ LARC offered first · ✓ EC hierarchy correct (CUP FIRST) · ✓ STI testing offered

✓ TRACE discussed · ✓ Inclusive language used · ✓ Safeguarding assessed (FORCED)

✓ PEP/PrEP recognised if indicated · ✓ FRAZER applied if under-16 · ✓ Safety-netting given

Final Exam Mantra

SAFER SEX → 5Ps + FORCED → UKMEC → LARC first → CUP FIRST → TRACE → OPEN → PEP/PrEP → FRAZER → ESCALATE

Gold Closing Statement:

"To summarise: I screened for pregnancy risk and safeguarding, assessed UKMEC safety, discussed contraception with LARC first, covered emergency contraception using CUP FIRST, offered STI testing with TRACE partner notification, addressed inclusive practice, considered HIV prevention where appropriate, and applied FRAZER guidelines if relevant. I know when to escalate immediately — including ectopic pregnancy, PID with sepsis, acute HIV, or safeguarding concerns."

SAFER SEX spine chapter framework	UKMEC 4 = no COC aura / breast cancer	CUP FIRST EC IUD > UPA > LNG	PEP <72 hours ideally <24h	LARC >99% fit and forget
5Ps + FORCED history + safeguarding	TRACE partner notification	OPEN language inclusive care	FRAZER <16 confidentiality assessment	Ectopic always positive test + pain

TOP 5 EXAMINER Q&A · WOMEN'S HEALTH I · CONTRACEPTION & SEXUAL HEALTH	
Q1. What is UKMEC and why does it matter?	The UK eligibility criteria grading contraceptive safety 1–4 against medical conditions; category 4 means do not use.
Q2. A 35-year-old smoker requests the combined pill?	UKMEC 4 if 35 or over and smoking 15 or more daily: offer progestogen-only or LARC alternatives.
Q3. Emergency contraception options and windows?	Copper IUD up to 5 days (most effective), ulipristal 120 hours, levonorgestrel 72 hours; discuss ongoing contraception.
Q4. What makes LARC first-line in counselling?	Highest effectiveness independent of user action; explain implant, IUS and IUD with typical-use failure rates.
Q5. How do you apply Fraser guidelines?	Under-16 contraception without parental consent if she understands, cannot be persuaded to inform parents, will continue intercourse, and her health is at risk; always assess safeguarding.
CURVEBALL	A 14-year-old requests contraception with an 18-year-old partner. Fraser competence is not the end of it: assess exploitation and safeguarding, and involve seniors per protocol.

CHAPTER 33 · WOMEN'S HEALTH II

Menopause & Antenatal Care

HRT · BABY CHECK · S.O.S · Pre-Eclampsia · RFM · MOVE Framework

VERY HIGH · CORE OSCE · CAUTION — HIGH INSTANT FAIL RISK

Abbreviations used in this chapter: **CBT** Cognitive Behavioural Therapy · **CTG** Cardiotocography · **GDM** Gestational Diabetes Mellitus · **HRT** Hormone Replacement Therapy · **ICP** Intracranial Pressure · **LMP** Last Menstrual Period · **RFM** Reduced Fetal Movements · **VTE** Venous Thromboembolism

Examiner Lens: "Can this doctor safely manage menopause and pregnancy, recognise red flags, and escalate appropriately with clear communication?"

Tested: Safe HRT decisions · Antenatal risk assessment · Pre-eclampsia prevention · RFM escalation · Safety-netting + communication

INSTANT FAIL Triggers:

HRT without checking contraindications · Postmenopausal bleeding ignored

Missed pre-eclampsia risk factors · No aspirin when indicated · Incomplete antenatal booking

RFM not escalated · Normal CTG but patient dismissed · No safety-netting

Instant Fail Reasoning Cards

Cognitive Error	Instant-Fail Behaviour	Saving Rule
Hearing "menopause" and treating the consultation as symptom control, so the bleeding history is never taken.	Starting or recommending HRT in a woman with undiagnosed vaginal bleeding.	Ask about bleeding before discussing HRT. Any postmenopausal or otherwise unexplained bleeding is investigated first — HRT waits. "Before we talk about treatment, I need to ask about any bleeding. If there's been any, we investigate that first — it changes what's safe to offer you."
Explaining bleeding that has already happened by the treatment or by atrophy, so it is never investigated.	Attributing postmenopausal bleeding to HRT or vaginal atrophy without urgent gynaecology referral for endometrial assessment.	Postmenopausal bleeding is cancer until proven otherwise — refer on the two-week-wait pathway for endometrial biopsy. "Any bleeding after the menopause needs to be investigated fully before we assume it's from the HRT or thinning of the lining. I'm referring you to the gynaecology team — they'll see you within two weeks."

Golden Opening · 8-Minute OSCE Structure

"Thank you for coming in. I'll ask a few questions to understand your symptoms or pregnancy, then we'll discuss safe options together so you can decide what feels right for you."

0–1 min	Opening
1–2 min	Focused history
2–3 min	Risk assessment
3–5 min	Explanation + options
5–6 min	Shared decision
6–7 min	Safety-net
7–8 min	Summary

PART A — MENOPAUSE

Core Symptoms · Always Rule Out

Core Symptoms	Always Rule Out
Hot flushes	Postmenopausal bleeding → urgent investigation BEFORE HRT
Night sweats	Unexplained weight loss
Mood change	Thyroid disorder
Vaginal dryness	
Reduced libido	

HRT — Safety Before Prescribing

Check before prescribing:
✓ Breast cancer history · ✓ VTE history · ✓ Unexplained bleeding · ✓ Liver disease · ✓ Uncontrolled hypertension

CAUTION — Migraine with aura → avoid oral HRT — use transdermal only.
CAUTION — Any persistent or new bleeding on HRT → needs investigation.

HRT Principle	Detail
Uterus present	Oestrogen + progesterone (combined HRT)
No uterus	Oestrogen-only
Risk factors present	Use transdermal route (not oral)
VTE/oral risk	Transdermal: no increased VTE vs oral

Non-HRT Options: SSRIs/SNRIs for flushes · Vaginal oestrogen for local symptoms · CBT + lifestyle · Specialist referral if complex

POI (<40 years): Refer to specialist · HRT needed for symptom + bone/heart protection until natural menopause age

PART B — ANTENATAL CARE

Antenatal Booking — BABY CHECK + S.O.S

BABY CHECK	Detail
Booking history	LMP · EDD · Gestation
Blood tests	FBC, blood group, rubella, Hep B, HIV, syphilis, Hep C
Blood pressure baseline	Mandatory at first visit
Medical + obstetric history	Previous pregnancies, complications, medical conditions
BMI	High BMI → pre-eclampsia risk + GDM screen
Family history	Genetic conditions, pre-eclampsia
Lifestyle + supplements	Folic acid + vitamin D · Alcohol · Smoking
Follow-up plan	Anomaly scan · Screening plan · Next appointment

S.O.S Safety Check:
S — Smoking/substances · O — Obstetric history · S — Safeguarding (ask alone)
SAY — Ask alone: "Are you feeling safe at home?"

Pre-Eclampsia Prevention

Risk Level	Risk Factors	Management
HIGH RISK	Previous pre-eclampsia · Kidney disease · Diabetes · Autoimmune disease	Low-dose aspirin — offer
MODERATE RISK	First pregnancy · High BMI · Age · Family history · Multiple pregnancy	≥2 moderate factors → aspirin
All indicated	Start early in pregnancy, continue until delivery	Regular BP + urine monitoring

Screening Overview: Early bloods · Anomaly scan (mid-pregnancy) · Growth monitoring if risk · GDM screen if indicated

Reduced Fetal Movements (RFM) — MOVE Framework

	MOVE	Action
M	Movement history	Frequency · pattern · last normal movement

	MOVE	Action
O	Observe fetal heart	Auscultation with Doppler
V	CTG if appropriate gestation	≥28 weeks → CTG
E	Escalate if concern	Maternal concern ALWAYS matters

Red Flags: Bleeding · Pain · No fetal heartbeat · Maternal concern
CAUTION — Key Principle: Normal CTG does NOT override ongoing maternal concern. If still worried → reassess or escalate.

Safety Netting · Must-Say Phrases

Return immediately if:
Reduced fetal movements persist · Bleeding or pain · Feeling unwell or worried · Sudden change in symptoms

Must-Say Phrases:
"We'll make a shared decision together." · "There is no single right answer."
"We will check safety before treatment."
"Please come back if you're worried — it's never a waste of time."

Examiner Checklist

Menopause	Antenatal	RFM
✓ Symptoms assessed	✓ BABY CHECK done	✓ MOVE used
✓ Contraindications checked	✓ Safeguarding (S.O.S)	✓ Fetal wellbeing assessed
✓ Safe HRT or alternatives	✓ Pre-eclampsia risk assessed	✓ Escalation appropriate
✓ Bleeding investigated	✓ Aspirin if indicated	✓ Maternal concern addressed
✓ Shared decision made	✓ Screening discussed	✓ Safety-net given

Final Exam Mantra

MENOPAUSE: Hot flush → Contraindications → Transdermal if risk → Investigate bleeding → Refer if persistent
ANTENATAL: BABY CHECK + S.O.S → Pre-eclampsia risk → Aspirin if indicated
RFM: MOVE → CTG if needed → Maternal concern ALWAYS matters
ALL: Safe → Explain → Document → Follow-up

Gold Closing Statement:
"We've discussed your symptoms/pregnancy, checked for safety, and gone through the options together. You understand the benefits and risks, and we've agreed on a plan that suits you. Please come back if anything changes or you're worried."

HRT contraindications check first always	PMB before HRT urgent investigation	Transdermal if risk migraine with aura rule	BABY CHECK structured booking	S.O.S safeguarding "are you safe at home?"
Aspirin 150mg daily in pregnancy (from 12 weeks) aspirin 150mg from 12 weeks (NICE NG133)	RFM = MOVE 4-step framework	Normal CTG does NOT override concern	Maternal concern always matters	Safety-net always "never a waste of time"

Intrahepatic Cholestasis of Pregnancy (ICP / Obstetric Cholestasis)

Presentation: Generalised itching in pregnancy (worse at night, palms and soles) · No rash (distinguishes from other causes) · Onset typically 2nd–3rd trimester · Jaundice rare but possible.

Investigations: LFTs (raised ALT/AST) · Serum bile acids (raised ≥10 μmol/L = diagnostic, ≥40 = high risk of stillbirth) · Clotting (impaired fat-soluble vitamin absorption).

Management: Ursodeoxycholic acid (UDCA) — reduces itch and improves bile acid levels · Increased fetal monitoring (CTG, growth scans) · Consider delivery at 37–38 weeks (higher risk of stillbirth if bile acids ≥40) · Vitamin K supplementation if prolonged clotting.

CAUTION — INSTANT FAIL: Reassuring a patient with itch in pregnancy without checking bile acids · Missing ICP as a cause of 3rd trimester itch · Failing to arrange increased fetal monitoring.

Must-Say: "I want to check your liver function tests and bile acid levels. Itching in pregnancy can be a sign of a liver condition that needs monitoring to keep your baby safe."

TOP 5 EXAMINER Q&A · WOMEN'S HEALTH II · MENOPAUSE & ANTENATAL CARE	
Q1. First-line treatment for vasomotor menopausal symptoms?	HRT after individualised risk-benefit discussion: combined if she has a uterus, oestrogen-only after hysterectomy.
Q2. Key HRT risks to counsel honestly?	Small increases in breast cancer (combined) and VTE (oral); transdermal avoids most VTE risk. Frame in absolute numbers.
Q3. Headache, visual disturbance and epigastric pain at 36 weeks?	Pre-eclampsia red flags: blood pressure and urine protein now, urgent obstetric review.
Q4. Reduced fetal movements. What is the rule?	Never reassure without assessment: same-day CTG and obstetric review every time.
Q5. Antenatal screening basics every candidate should state?	Booking bloods, anomaly scans, gestational diabetes risk assessment and blood pressure/urine at every contact.

TOP 5 EXAMINER Q&A · WOMEN'S HEALTH II · MENOPAUSE & ANTENATAL CARE	
CURVEBALL	She read that HRT "causes cancer" and refuses all options. Explore the fear, give absolute risks both ways, offer alternatives, and respect an informed choice: document the discussion.

CHAPTER 34 · LIFESTYLE MEDICINE

Smoking Cessation & Weight Management

CORE · CAUTION — HIGH INSTANT FAIL RISK · SAY — COMMUNICATION-HEAVY

Abbreviations used in this chapter: NRT Nicotine Replacement Therapy

Why This Chapter:

These stations test: building rapport quickly · avoiding judgement · exploring readiness for change · giving safe options · agreeing realistic goals · ensuring follow-up

THINK — Core Principle: Behaviour change only works when the patient feels in control of the decision.

Examiners REWARD: Calm, non-judgemental · Respects autonomy · Explores motivation · Safe prescribing awareness · Small realistic goals · Clear follow-up

Examiners do NOT reward: Long explanations · Medical complexity · Announcing frameworks · Excessive detail

Instant Fail Triggers

Judgemental or shaming language · Starting advice without permission · Ignoring patient readiness

No shared decision-making · Unsafe smoking advice in pregnancy · Missing mood warning for varenicline

Overloading with medical detail · No follow-up or safety net · Pushing change too strongly in unready patient

TIP — Overall Consultation Flow — Use Invisibly

1. Permission + opening → 2. Explore experience and motivation → 3. Offer simple options safely → 4. Agree one small change → 5. Plan follow-up and support

(Do NOT announce this structure to the patient)

PART A — SMOKING CESSATION

SAY — Smoking — Consultation Scripts

Stage	Script
Opening (ask permission)	"Would it be okay if we talk about your smoking today?" · "If not, we can focus on what's most important for you."
Explore experience	"What do you enjoy about smoking?" · "Have you thought about stopping before?" · "What makes it difficult?"
Reflect	"So it helps with stress, but you're also worried about your health."
Offer help	"If you're open to it, I can talk you through a few options."
Agree plan	"What feels like a realistic first step for you?" Examples: set a quit date · start patches · reduce gradually
Check confidence	"On a scale of 0–10, how confident do you feel about that?" If low: "What would help make it more achievable?"

Stage	Script
Follow-up	Review in 1–2 weeks · Normalise relapse: "If things don't go perfectly, that's very normal. We can adjust together."

Smoking Options — NRT · Varenicline · Vaping

Option	Detail	Key Safety Point
NRT Patch	Steady nicotine level · Usually 8–12 weeks then reduce	Safe first-line · Combination more effective for heavier smokers
NRT Gum/Spray	Helps sudden cravings	Use alongside patch for combination approach
Varenicline	Most effective medication for smoking cessation	Mood changes warning: low mood / suicidal thoughts → stop immediately and seek help
Vaping	Less harmful than smoking · Not risk-free	Aim: fully switch, not use both
Pregnancy	Behavioural support first	NRT safer than continuing smoking · Much safer for baby

Varenicline Caution: History of mental illness · Seizures · Kidney problems — review before prescribing

PART B — WEIGHT MANAGEMENT

SAY — Weight Management — Consultation Scripts

Stage	Script
Opening (ask permission)	"Would it be okay if we talk about your weight in relation to your health?"
Explore context	Diet patterns · Activity level · Stress and emotional eating · Social or financial barriers
Reflect	"It sounds like it's been quite difficult to manage with everything going on."
Simple advice	Focus on health, not appearance · Small sustainable changes · "Even reducing sugary drinks can make a difference."
Agree one small step	"What's one small change you feel you could try this week?" Examples: 20-min walk · swap sugary drinks · smaller portions
Check confidence	"How confident are you about doing that?"
Follow-up	Review in 4–6 weeks · "We'll review progress and adjust if needed — this is a gradual process."

Weight Red Flags + Support Options

Be alert for:
Rapid weight change · Eating disorder behaviour · Thyroid or Cushing's symptoms · PCOS features · Psychological distress affecting eating
If suspected: "I'd like to check for any underlying medical or psychological causes as well."

Support Options:
Dietitian referral · Structured weight management services · Social prescribing · Mental health support if needed

Key Communication Skills — Hidden Marking Area

✓ Do	SAY — High-Yield Phrase
Ask permission before advice	"Would it be okay if we talk about this?"
Reflect patient feelings	"So it sounds like…"
Avoid judgement	"I understand this has been difficult."
Normalise ambivalence	"Many people feel mixed about this."
Avoid pressure to change	"This is your decision."
Focus on one priority	Agree one small step only
Shared decision-making	"What feels realistic for you?"
Relapse frame	"Relapse is very common and does not mean failure."

Examiner Checklist

✓ Permission obtained · ✓ Non-judgemental tone · ✓ Patient concerns explored
✓ Safe options offered · ✓ Shared decision-making used · ✓ Smoking advice correct (NRT + varenicline + vaping)
✓ Pregnancy advice correct · ✓ Weight red flags considered · ✓ Realistic plan agreed
✓ Follow-up arranged · ✓ Safety net given · ✓ Relapse normalised

Final Exam Mantra

Permission → Explore → Offer options → Agree one small step → Follow up

Gold Closing Statement:
"To summarise, we've talked about your situation, explored options, and agreed a small realistic step. We'll review how things are going and adjust the plan if needed. You're not expected to do everything at once — this is a gradual process."

Ask permission first every time, every station	Never shame non-judgemental always	Explore readiness before any advice	NRT first-line 8–12 weeks	Varenicline mood warning stop + seek help
Pregnancy NRT safe safer than smoking	One small step not everything at once	Relapse is normal adjust plan together	Weight red flags eating disorder + thyroid	Follow-up always review + adjust

TOP 5 EXAMINER Q&A · LIFESTYLE MEDICINE	
Q1. Most effective single smoking-cessation strategy?	Behavioural support combined with pharmacotherapy: varenicline or combination NRT; offer at every contact.
Q2. How do you open a weight conversation without harm?	Ask permission first: “Would it be okay to talk about weight today?”; avoid blame and focus on health goals.
Q3. What are the alcohol screening steps?	AUDIT-C then full AUDIT if positive; brief intervention for hazardous drinking, specialist referral for dependence.
Q4. Safe drinking guidance in the UK?	No more than 14 units a week for men and women, spread over 3 or more days, with drink-free days.
Q5. Exercise prescription basics?	150 minutes of moderate activity weekly plus strength work twice a week, adapted to the individual’s starting point.
CURVEBALL	“I’ve tried everything and nothing works.” Validate the frustration, explore what was actually tried, and agree one small specific achievable change: success builds on success.

CHAPTER 35 · COMMON PRESENTATIONS

Shingles · Red Leg · Eczema/Psoriasis · Skin Cancer · Red Eye · ENT Emergencies

HIGH YIELD · GP / Minor Injuries / ED · CAUTION — MODERATE INSTANT FAIL RISK

ESCALATION UNDER UNCERTAINTY

Abbreviations used in this chapter: **DVT** Deep Vein Thrombosis · **FTU** Fingertip Unit · **PE** Pulmonary Embolism · **USS** Ultrasound Scan

Core Exam Purpose:

You are NOT tested on diagnosis. You are tested on: Can you recognise danger early and escalate immediately under uncertainty?

THINK — Examiner Thinking: "Would I feel safe leaving this patient with this doctor right now?"

Global Safety Principle: Always treat loss of function (vision, breathing, limb swelling, acute severe pain) as urgent until proven otherwise.

High Scoring: Early escalation · Worst-case thinking · Clear safety language · No hesitation on red flags

Instant Fail Triggers

Situation	Immediate Action
Stridor	CALL SENIOR + ANAESTHETICS — DO NOT examine throat
Painful red eye + vision loss	SAME-DAY OPHTHALMOLOGY
Suspected melanoma	2-WEEK WAIT (2WW) REFERRAL
DVT likely (Wells ≥2)	ANTICOAGULATE + URGENT USS
Shingles + nose tip (Hutchinson's)	SAME-DAY OPHTHALMOLOGY
Orbital cellulitis	ADMIT IV ANTIBIOTICS

Station Recognition:

Itchy scaly rash → Eczema/Psoriasis · Red hot swollen leg → Cellulitis vs DVT · Dermatomal vesicles → Shingles

Changing mole → Skin cancer · Red painful eye → Emergency until proven otherwise · Stridor/drooling → Airway emergency

Shingles — Hutchinson's Sign

Pattern: Unilateral burning pain → vesicles → DOES NOT cross midline

Hutchinson's Sign: Tip/side of nose involvement → nasociliary nerve → eye at risk → SAME-DAY ophthalmology even if asymptomatic.

SAY — Must-Say: "Because the rash involves the nerve connected to your eye, you need urgent eye assessment today even if your eye feels fine."

Management	Detail
Antivirals	≥72h from rash onset ideally
After 72h: give if…	New vesicles appear OR ophthalmic involvement suspected OR immunocompromised
Analgesia	Early, adequate
Self-care	Keep rash clean/dry · Avoid vulnerable contacts (pregnant, immunocompromised)
Complication	Post-herpetic neuralgia — risk increases with age + severity

Red Leg — Cellulitis vs DVT vs Lymphoedema

Feature	Cellulitis	DVT	Lymphoedema
Onset	Acute	Acute/subacute	Chronic
Pain	Tender, hot	Deep calf pain	Painless
Swelling	Localised	Whole limb	Diffuse
Fever	Common	Rare	No

THINK — Core Rule: Always rule out DVT before confirming infection.
SAY — Must-Say: "We need to rule out a clot as well as infection."

Diagnosis	Management
Cellulitis	Antibiotics · Mark margin (exam tick-box) · Review 48h
DVT (Wells ≥2)	Anticoagulate immediately · Urgent USS · Bleeding risk check · Explain PE red flags: chest pain, breathlessness, haemoptysis
Lymphoedema	Compression + elevation + referral
Sepsis trigger	Fever + tachycardia + confusion + hypotension → Escalate immediately

Eczema · Psoriasis

Condition	Stepwise Management	Key Safety Point
Eczema	1. Emollients (daily, always) 2. Mild steroids (face/flexures) 3. Potent steroids (body, short bursts) 4. Treat infection if present	FTU rule: 1 fingertip unit = 2 adult palms
Eczema Herpeticum	Pain out of proportion (KEY CLUE) + widespread vesicles + fever	ADMIT IMMEDIATELY + IV aciclovir

Condition	Stepwise Management	Key Safety Point
Psoriasis	Emollients → Vitamin D analogues → Potent steroids → Phototherapy → Systemic (specialist)	Systemic = specialist only

SAY — Eczema Must-Say: "Use emollients daily and steroids only during flares in short controlled bursts."

Skin Cancer — ABCDE + Referral Rules

ABCDE: Asymmetry · Border · Colour · Diameter >6mm · Evolution

Condition	Action
Melanoma / SCC / Nodular melanoma	2WW URGENT REFERRAL
Immunosuppressed + changing lesion	2WW URGENT REFERRAL
BCC	Routine referral (unless high-risk site)

SAY — Must-Say: "This needs urgent assessment under the 2-week cancer pathway."

Red Eye — High-Risk Until Proven Otherwise

Red Flags: Pain · Vision loss · Photophobia · Irregular pupil · Deep pain · Contact lens use · Ciliary flush · Corneal opacity

Contact Lens Rule: Stop immediately → assume microbial keratitis until proven otherwise.

Condition	Action
Conjunctivitis	Drops · hygiene advice
Iritis	Ophthalmology
Acute angle closure	Emergency
Scleritis	Referral
Corneal abrasion	Antibiotics · lubricants
Herpes keratitis	NO STEROIDS — antiviral only
Chemical injury	Immediate irrigation + ophthalmology
Endophthalmitis	Emergency

SAY — Must-Say: "Because your vision is affected, this needs urgent specialist assessment today."

Orbital vs Preseptal Cellulitis:
Preseptal: Normal eye movement · normal vision · no proptosis → Oral antibiotics
Orbital: Restricted movement · reduced vision · proptosis → ADMIT + IV antibiotics + ophthalmology
SAY — Must-Say: "This is orbital cellulitis — this is a hospital emergency requiring IV antibiotics."

ENT Emergencies

Stridor Rule: DO NOT examine throat · CALL senior + anaesthetics immediately · NO imaging delay if airway risk suspected.
SAY — Must-Say: "This is an airway emergency — I'm calling anaesthetics immediately."

Condition	Action
Quinsy	ENT drainage + IV antibiotics
Perichondritis	Ciprofloxacin (lobule spared — differentiates from otitis externa)
Epistaxis	Pressure → Naseptin (check peanut allergy)
Button battery	IMMEDIATE removal — no delay for imaging

CAUTION — Naseptin contains peanut oil — always check allergy before prescribing.

High-Yield Numbers · Communication · Safety-Net

Key Number/Rule	Detail
Shingles antivirals	Start ≤72h ideally (exceptions apply after 72h)
Cellulitis review	48 hours
DVT threshold	Wells ≥2 → anticoagulate
Cancer referral	2WW (2-week wait)
FTU eczema	1 fingertip unit = 2 adult palms

Communication (Exam Scoring Zone):
"Would it be okay to talk about this today?"
"Let me check I've explained this clearly — what are your main concerns?"
"This could be infection or a clot — I need to rule out clot urgently."
"Because your vision is affected, this needs urgent assessment."
Never Say: "It's probably nothing" · "Don't worry" · "You are obese" · Framework names out loud

Safety-Net (Mandatory):
"If symptoms worsen, pain increases, you develop fever, or your vision changes — seek urgent medical help immediately."

Final Exam Mantra

Red flags first. · Act in uncertainty. · Escalate early. · Speak simply. · Safety-net every time.

Gold Closing Statement:
"We've discussed your condition today. This is likely [X]. We are going to [Y]. If [Z happens], seek urgent help immediately. Do you have any questions?"

Stridor call anaesthetics — no throat exam	Hutchinson's sign same-day ophthalmology	DVT Wells ≥2 anticoagulate + USS	Rule out DVT first before confirming cellulitis	Melanoma 2WW urgent referral
Herpes keratitis no steroids ever	Orbital cellulitis admit IV antibiotics	Eczema herpeticum admit IV aciclovir	Button battery immediate removal	Safety-net always every single station

TOP 5 EXAMINER Q&A · COMMON PRESENTATIONS	
Q1. Shingles management and the time rule?	Aciclovir within 72 hours of rash onset if eligible; urgent ophthalmology if the eye or nose tip is involved.
Q2. Unilateral red hot swollen leg: cellulitis or DVT?	They can coexist; use Wells scoring and have a low threshold for D-dimer/ultrasound rather than anchoring on cellulitis.
Q3. Red flags in a "simple rash" station?	Non-blanching purpura, mucosal involvement, skin pain out of proportion, systemic toxicity: think meningococcus, SJS, necrotising infection.
Q4. Which moles need two-week-wait referral?	Use the weighted 7-point checklist: change in size, shape or colour score highest; if in doubt, refer.
Q5. The dangerous red eye features?	Pain (not grittiness), photophobia, reduced acuity, fixed pupil: same-day ophthalmology.
CURVEBALL	A "cellulitis" that is exquisitely painful beyond findings, with crepitus. Necrotising fasciitis until excluded: IV antibiotics and immediate surgical review.

CHAPTER 36 · LONG-TERM CONDITION REVIEWS

CKD · Liver · Thyroid · Osteoporosis · Travel

HIGH YIELD · GP / Outpatient · CAUTION — HIGH INSTANT FAIL RISK

Abbreviations used in this chapter: **CKD** Chronic Kidney Disease · **DVT** Deep Vein Thrombosis · **PE** Pulmonary Embolism · **SBP** Systolic Blood Pressure

Instant Fail Reasoning Cards

Cognitive Error	Instant-Fail Behaviour	Saving Rule
Treating a long-term condition review as a consultation about whatever the patient raised.	Completing the review and closing the consultation without measuring blood pressure.	Measure blood pressure in every long-term condition review, before closing, regardless of what the patient came in to discuss. "Before we finish, I'm going to check your blood pressure — that's part of every review."
Treating the review as a data-collection exercise rather than a decision point.	Documenting an abnormal result — CKD stage, HbA1c, blood pressure — during the review and neither acting on it nor arranging follow-up.	An abnormal result must change management: escalate, adjust treatment, or bring the review forward. Do not document and move on. "This result is outside the normal range, so we can't just file it. I'm going to change your treatment today and bring your next review forward — we need a plan for this now."
Reading new symptoms in a known long-term condition as more of the same condition.	Discharging a patient from a review who has new or worsening symptoms without investigating the cause or arranging follow-up.	New symptoms in a long-term condition patient are not "just the condition" — consider acute deterioration, complication or new pathology, and investigate. "You've had this condition for years, but these symptoms are new for you. That means we need to check whether something has changed — it could be a complication, a new problem, or a deterioration. I'm not going to assume it's just the condition."

Core Exam Theme: You are tested on: "Can this doctor monitor safely, detect deterioration early, and escalate without delay?"

Universal Pass Behaviour: Stage disease correctly · Detect deterioration early · Escalate before certainty · Stop harmful drugs · Safety-net · Worst-case first

CAUTION — Global Clinical Rule: If two diagnoses are possible and one is dangerous → manage as dangerous until excluded.

Global Safety Triage — Always treat as urgent:
Loss of function (vision/breathing/consciousness/mobility) · Sepsis features · Suspected DVT/PE
Acute confusion · End-organ decompensation (liver/renal/endocrine crisis)

CKD Review — Safe + Complete

Must Do: eGFR stage (G1–G5) · ACR category (A1–A3) · BP + CV risk · Medication review

ACEi/ARB Monitoring	Detail
Before starting	Check U&Es
After starting/dose change	Repeat U&Es at 1–2 weeks
Ongoing	At least annually
STOP if	K^+ >5.5 mmol/L OR Creatinine rise >30%

Also consider: Stop NSAIDs (nephrotoxic) · Assess dehydration risk · Review diuretics
SADMAN — Sick Day Rules:
S — SGLT2i · A — ACEi · D — Diuretics · M — Metformin · A — ARBs · N — NSAIDs
Stop during: vomiting/diarrhoea/fever. Restart after 24h normal intake.
SAY — Must-Say: "If you become unwell with vomiting, diarrhoea, or fever, temporarily stop these medicines to protect your kidneys."

Liver Disease — Decompensation System

Red Flags → ADMIT:
Confusion (encephalopathy) · GI bleeding · Fever + ascites · Worsening jaundice · Rising creatinine
SAY — Must-Say: "Confusion in liver disease is an emergency — this needs hospital assessment today."

	LIVER Framework	Detail
L	Lethargy (encephalopathy)	Check asterixis (flapping tremor)
I	Icterus	LFTs · bilirubin · INR
V	Varices	EMERGENCY bleed — resuscitate + terlipressin + endoscopy
E	Oedema / ascites	Spironolactone + furosemide
R	Risk of SBP	Ascitic neutrophils >250 → IV antibiotics + albumin immediately

SBP Rule: Ascitic neutrophils >250 → IV antibiotics immediately + IV albumin. Send ascitic culture before antibiotics if possible — but DO NOT delay treatment.
Also consider: Hepatorenal syndrome if rising creatinine without cause · Infection = most common trigger of encephalopathy · Do not discharge confused cirrhotic patients

Thyroid Emergencies — Storm vs Myxoedema Coma

Feature	Thyroid Storm	Myxoedema Coma
Temperature	HIGH (hyperpyrexia)	LOW (hypothermia)
Heart rate	Fast (tachycardia)	Slow (bradycardia)
Mental state	Agitated	Coma / confused
Skin	Warm, sweaty	Cold, dry

Condition	Management
Thyroid Storm	Beta-blocker · Carbimazole/PTU FIRST · Steroids · Iodine ≥1 hour AFTER antithyroid (minimum 1h; some protocols recommend longer) · Treat trigger · Burch-Wartofsky >45 = storm
Myxoedema Coma	ICU · IV T4 (levothyroxine) FIRST · Hydrocortisone (adrenal cover) · Slow rewarming · Correct hyponatraemia slowly · T3 only if severe/non-responsive

SAY — Must-Say: “Both are life-threatening endocrine emergencies requiring hospital admission.”

Osteoporosis — BONES Counselling

Diagnosis: T-score ≤−2.5 = osteoporosis · Fragility fracture = treat regardless · FRAX above threshold = treat

	BONES Counselling	Detail
B	Be aware (fracture prevention)	Home hazard assessment
O	On empty stomach	Take bisphosphonate on empty stomach
N	No food 30–60 min	Stay upright after taking
E	Erect (30 min upright)	Prevent oesophageal irritation
S	Supplements (Ca + Vit D)	Co-prescribe with bisphosphonates

Key Safety Step: Dental check BEFORE bisphosphonates · Ask about jaw problems / dental issues (osteonecrosis risk)

Drug Holiday: Oral bisphosphonate: 5 years → reassess. Stop if low risk. Monitor every 2–3 years.

Screen secondary causes if early/severe: Thyroid disease · Coeliac · Myeloma · Steroid use · Hypogonadism

SAY — Must-Say: “This strengthens bones and reduces fracture risk, but we need a dental check before starting.”

Travel Medicine — Safe + Complete

First Step — Check Before Vaccines:
Pregnancy? · Immunosuppression? → determines LIVE vaccine safety

Category	Vaccines	Key Safety Points
LIVE (caution)	Yellow fever · Oral typhoid CAUTION — Yellow fever is the ONLY travel vaccine that cannot be given in pregnancy. Hepatitis A, typhoid (inactivated injectable), and meningococcal vaccines are inactivated and safe in pregnancy.	Avoid in pregnancy + immunosuppression
Non-live (safe)	Hep A · Hep B · Tetanus · Rabies · Meningococcal ACWY	Safe in most groups
Malaria prophylaxis	Atovaquone-proguanil (first line)	ALWAYS include bite prevention: DEET + nets + clothing — MOST IMPORTANT
Mefloquine — screen	Check before prescribing	Depression · Anxiety · Psychosis · Epilepsy → AVOID

SAY — Must-Say: "Vaccines should ideally be given 4–6 weeks before travel to ensure protection."

Universal Red Flags · Communication · Safety-Net

Universal Red Flags:
Stridor → airway emergency · Vision loss + red eye → urgent ophthalmology
DVT suspected → anticoagulate · Sepsis signs → immediate escalation
Confusion in liver disease → admit · Neuro deficit → urgent imaging

Communication Markers:
"Let me check I've explained this clearly — what would you do if things worsen?"
"This could be serious, so I want to be safe and investigate urgently."
"We need hospital assessment today to rule out dangerous causes."
Never say: "It's probably nothing" · "Don't worry" · Unqualified reassurance

Global Safety-Net (Mandatory):
"If symptoms worsen, or you develop fever, confusion, breathlessness, chest pain, or vision changes — seek urgent medical help immediately."

Final Exam Mantra

Recognise risk early. · Think worst-case first. · Escalate without delay. · Speak simply. · Safety-net every time.

Gold OSCE Closing:
"We've reviewed your condition today. You have [condition]. We will [plan]. This is to keep you safe and prevent complications. If anything worsens, seek urgent help immediately. Do you have any questions?"

CKD SADMAN stop in illness	ACEi stop if K+ >5.5 or Cr rise >30%	SBP rule neutrophils >250 → IV Abx	Liver confusion emergency admit	Storm vs myxoedema hot/fast vs cold/slow
Iodine timing 1h after antithyroid	Dental check first before bisphosphonates	BONES framework bisphosphonate counselling	Live vaccines CAUTION — Yellow fever = ONLY travel vaccine contraindicated in pregnancy. Hep A/typhoid (inactivated) safe in pregnancy.	Mefloquine screen depression/psychosis/epilepsy

TOP 5 EXAMINER Q&A · LONG-TERM CONDITION REVIEWS	
Q1. How is CKD staged and monitored?	By eGFR category and urine ACR; the ACR predicts progression: check both at every review.
Q2. When does CKD need nephrology referral?	ACR 70 or more, eGFR below 30, rapid decline, or resistant hypertension: refer per NICE criteria.
Q3. Abnormal LFTs in primary care: first steps?	History (alcohol, drugs, metabolic risk), liver screen bloods and ultrasound; calculate a fibrosis score before referral.
Q4. Starting levothyroxine: how do you monitor?	Recheck TSH at 6–8 weeks after any dose change, then annually once stable.
Q5. Who gets a FRAX assessment?	Women 65 and over, men 75 and over, or younger with risk factors; treat or DXA according to the result.
CURVEBALL	Three long-term conditions, twelve medications, one 10-minute review. Prioritise with the patient: ask what matters most to them today: that is the consultation the examiner wants.

CHAPTER 37 · THE FRAIL OLDER PATIENT

Safety-Led Frailty Assessment · System Failure State, Not Diagnosis

FRAILTY CGA · PINCH ME · FALLS SAFE · STOPP/START · URWC · MDT

VERY HIGH · GP / COE / Acute Take / Home Visit · CAUTION — HIGH INSTANT FAIL RISK

Abbreviations used in this chapter: AMTS Abbreviated Mental Test Score · **CGA** Comprehensive Geriatric Assessment · **MDT** Multidisciplinary Team

Core Exam Focus: Safe decision-making in physiological vulnerability

✓ Recognise frailty as high-risk system state · ✓ Identify multifactorial causes (NEVER single-cause falls)

✓ Detect delirium early · ✓ Manage polypharmacy safely · ✓ Assess capacity (decision-specific, fluctuating)

Examiner Lens: "Does this doctor prevent avoidable harm while preserving independence safely?"

Candidate ALWAYS: Establishes baseline first · Treats falls as multifactorial · Rules out delirium before dementia · Includes carer

Instant Fail

"Mechanical fall" without assessment · No postural BP · No medication review

Misses delirium / calls it dementia · No 4AT · Misses hypoactive delirium

No head injury check in anticoagulated patient · No gait assessment · No bladder scan

No capacity assessment · Unsafe discharge without home assessment · Ignores carer concerns

Station Recognition · Golden Minute

Trigger	Likely Problem
"Had a fall"	Multifactorial fall + postural hypotension
"Confused / off baseline"	Delirium until proven otherwise
"On many tablets"	Polypharmacy harm
"Not coping at home"	Carer strain / safeguarding
"Off legs"	Infection / fracture / dehydration / frailty collapse

SAY — Golden Minute Opening:

"This is a frail older adult with reduced physiological reserve. I will first establish baseline function and recent changes. I am concerned about multifactorial causes including falls, delirium, medication effects, and functional decline. I will assess reversible causes early, involve the carer, and ensure safe disposition planning."

THINK — Frailty CGA Framework — FRAILY (Autopilot System)

	FRAILY	Actions	Fail if Missed
F	FALLS (always multifactorial)	Postural BP · Gait · ECG if syncope · Head injury check	Missing postural BP
R	R — Review (Medications)	"Any recent medication changes?" · STOPP/START · Anticholinergics · Antihypertensives	No medication review
A	A — Assessment (Cognition: Delirium vs Dementia)	4AT · Acute+fluctuating+inattention=delirium · Hypoactive delirium · Collateral history Tool distinction: 4AT = use for DELIRIUM screening (acute, fluctuating change). AMTS = use for BASELINE COGNITION in a stable patient. Do not use AMTS alone when delirium is possible.	Calling delirium dementia
I	I — Integration (Carer System)	"How are YOU coping?" · Carer strain = patient risk marker · Support/respite	Ignoring carer concerns
L	L — Levels of risk (Safeguarding)	Neglect/self-neglect · Fearful behaviour · Unexplained injury · "Do you feel safe at home?"	Missing safeguarding
Y	Y — Your baseline (Functional)	ADLs · Mobility baseline · Vision + hearing · Nutrition	No baseline established

Delirium — PINCH ME (Medical Emergency)

THINK — "Delirium is a medical emergency until proven otherwise." · "Hypoactive delirium can be missed."

P	Pain	Unrecognised pain — especially post-fall
I	Infection	UTI, chest, skin, urosepsis
N	Nutrition / Dehydration	Acute dehydration common in frailty
C	Constipation / Urinary retention	Bladder scan mandatory
H	Hypoxia	SpO_2 + RR
M	Medications	Anticholinergics, opioids, benzodiazepines
E	Electrolytes / Environment	Na/Ca/glucose · unfamiliar environment worsens delirium

ABCDE — Frailty Adaptation

A	Airway	↓ consciousness → escalate immediately
B	Breathing	Hypoxia / infection → delirium
C	Circulation	Postural BP + dehydration
D	Disability	4AT + glucose + bladder scan
E	Exposure	Trauma / infection / safeguarding

"New inability to walk is an emergency until proven otherwise."

Falls System — FALLS SAFE

F	Footwear	Check suitability
A	Antihypertensives	Postural hypotension risk
L	Lighting	Especially nocturnal
L	Leg weakness	Physiotherapy referral
S	Sedatives	Benzodiazepines/Z-drugs
S	Sensory loss	Vision + hearing
A	Acute illness	UTI/chest/dehydration
F	Floor hazards	Loose rugs, cables
E	Environment (OT home review)	Mandatory before discharge

Polypharmacy — STOPP/START

STOPP (Consider stopping)	**✓ START (Consider starting)**
Benzodiazepines / Z-drugs	Vitamin D ± calcium
Anticholinergics	Osteoporosis prevention if indicated
NSAIDs (renal/GI risk)	
Long-term PPIs (unnecessary)	
Hypotensive antihypertensives	
Alpha blockers	

Rules: One change at a time · Check renal function · Shared decision-making · Avoid abrupt withdrawal · "Any recent medication changes?" = Gold Question

Capacity (URWC) · Discharge vs Admission

URWC: Understand · Retain · Weigh · Communicate — Decision-specific · Fluctuates in delirium · Assume capacity first · Maximise communication

Safe Discharge Only If	Admission Triggers
Safe mobility (OT/PT cleared)	Delirium + unsafe home
Home environment safe	New inability to mobilise
Medication plan safe	Suspected fracture
Carer coping confirmed	Safeguarding concern
Capacity documented	Carer breakdown
Follow-up arranged	

Examiner Checklist — SSE Structured Summary

✓ Baseline established first · ✓ Falls multifactorial + postural BP + gait
✓ Delirium assessed (4AT + PINCH ME) · ✓ Medication risk reviewed (STOPP/START)
✓ Carer involved and assessed · ✓ Safeguarding considered ("Do you feel safe?")
✓ Safe discharge decision made · ✓ MDT input documented · ✓ Capacity assessed

Final Exam Mantra

"There is no such thing as a simple mechanical fall."
"Delirium is always acute and fluctuating." · "Hypoactive delirium can be missed."
"Every medication is a potential cause until reviewed."
"Capacity is decision-specific." · "I will only discharge if the home is safe."

Gold Closing Statement:
"This is a frail older adult with high physiological vulnerability. My assessment focused on baseline function, reversible causes, cognition, medications, and home safety. The most likely issue is multifactorial frailty with contributions such as delirium, postural hypotension, medication effects, or infection. I have addressed reversible risks and involved the MDT. I will ensure discharge only if the home environment is safe with adequate support."

Baseline first critical anchor	No mechanical falls always multifactorial	Postural BP mandatory every frailty station	4AT + PINCH ME delirium assessment	Hypoactive delirium actively consider
STOPP/START polypharmacy safety	"Any med changes?" gold question	FALLS SAFE 9-component screen	Carer strain patient risk marker	OT home review before every discharge

TOP 5 EXAMINER Q&A · THE FRAIL OLDER PATIENT	
Q1. What is comprehensive geriatric assessment?	Multidimensional MDT review of medical, functional, psychological and social domains producing a coordinated plan.
Q2. Key components of a falls assessment?	History of falls, medication review, lying-standing blood pressure, gait and balance, vision, bone health and home hazards.

TOP 5 EXAMINER Q&A · THE FRAIL OLDER PATIENT	
Q3. What are STOPP/START criteria for?	Identifying potentially inappropriate prescriptions to stop and indicated treatments to start in older adults.
Q4. How do you assess capacity in cognitive impairment?	Decision-specific: understand, retain, weigh and communicate; impairment does not equal incapacity.
Q5. Anticholinergic burden: why care?	Cumulative anticholinergic load drives confusion, falls and mortality: count it and deprescribe.
CURVEBALL	The family insists “she must go to a home” but the patient with capacity refuses. Her capacitous decision stands: arrange support, manage risk, and document: autonomy is not negotiable.

CHAPTER 38 · EATING DISORDERS & ACUTE MEDICAL RISK

NOT A THERAPY STATION — THIS IS ACUTE MEDICAL ADMISSION DECISION

13-40-90 · MEED · SUSS · Refeeding · QTc · Phosphate · SBAR · MDT

VERY HIGH · RED PATH · CAUTION — CRITICAL INSTANT FAIL RISK

Abbreviations used in this chapter: **MDT** Multidisciplinary Team · **SBP** Systolic Blood Pressure

THINK — Core Exam Truth: Eating disorders = silent physiological collapse until proven otherwise.

Examiner Lens: "Does this candidate detect hidden medical instability and escalate BEFORE deterioration?"

You pass ONLY if you: Use objective instability (not reassurance) · Admit early · Prevent refeeding complications · Escalate (SBAR + MDT)

Instant Fail

Discharge with unstable vitals · Psychiatry before medical stabilisation · No ECG / ignores QTc

No phosphate monitoring · No thiamine before feeding · Misses hypoglycaemia ("feels fine")

Ignores purging → hypokalaemia · No SBAR · No MDT · Wrong BMI system in <18

Admission Decision Engine — ANY ONE TRIGGER = ADMIT

13-40-90 Rule:

BMI <13 (or <70% centile if <18) · HR <40 bpm · SBP <90 OR postural drop >20 mmHg

MEED — Parameter	Threshold
QTc	>450 ms (male) / >460 ms (female) — >500 ms = emergency
K^+	<3.0 mmol/L
Phosphate (PO_4)	<0.8 mmol/L
Glucose	<3.0 mmol/L
SUSS test	Fail (cannot squat-stand without arms) = muscle + cardiac reserve depletion
Rapid weight loss	>1 kg/week
Syncope/collapse	Any episode

Final Rule: ANY ONE = MEDICAL ADMISSION (non-negotiable). Uncertainty = ADMIT + ESCALATE.

Station Recognition — Pattern Lock

"I don't eat much" → Starvation physiology · "I feel fine" → Silent collapse risk · Collapse → Arrhythmia until proven otherwise
Vomiting/laxatives → Electrolyte depletion · Low BMI → MEED until excluded
Must-Say Opening: "This is medical stabilisation, not therapy." · "Physical safety is the priority."

OSCE Execution Flow

Phase	Time	Action
Safety scan	0–60 sec	ABCDE · Glucose · HR/BP/temp · Confusion = red flag → instability = ADMIT mindset immediately
Risk confirm	1–3 min	Weight/BMI or centile · restriction duration · purging/laxatives · collapse history
Investigations	3–5 min	ECG → QTc · U&E · PHOSPHATE · Magnesium · Glucose
Decision	5–6 min	IF ANY ONE TRIGGER → ADMIT
Action	6–8 min	Medical admission · cardiac monitor if QTc risk · correct electrolytes · thiamine BEFORE feeding · SBAR + MDT

ECG Rule · Silent Hypoglycaemia · SUSS Test

ECG Rule: QTc >450 ms (M) / >460 ms (F) = risk · QTc >500 ms = emergency
Avoid: Citalopram · Haloperidol · Macrolides · Ondansetron (QT-prolonging)

Silent Hypoglycaemia (High-Yield Trap): Glucose <3.0 + asymptomatic — MUST NOT WALK → trolley only.
Order: 1. Confirm glucose · 2. Pabrinex BEFORE glucose · 3. Give glucose/food · 4. Recheck glucose · 5. ECG if needed

SUSS Test: Sit → Squat → Stand without hands. FAIL = global muscle + cardiac reserve depletion.

Refeeding Syndrome Prevention

Mechanism: Starvation → insulin surge on refeeding → phosphate shift into cells → hypophosphataemia → arrhythmia/cardiac failure

Action	Detail
Thiamine BEFORE feeding	Pabrinex IV — non-negotiable
Start low calorie	5–10 kcal/kg/24h initially
Daily phosphate	Days 3–5 = peak risk period
Replace electrolytes	K^+ / PO_4 / Magnesium proactively
Slow escalation	Dietitian-led · "Nutrition = controlled medical therapy"

Disposition · MDT · Under-18 Rules

Admit if Any of These	MDT Team	Under-18 Rules
MEED positive	Medical registrar — admission decision	BMI centiles only (NOT absolute)
Abnormal ECG	Dietitian — refeeding plan	<70% median for age = admission
Electrolyte abnormality	Psychiatry — after medical stable	Paeds + CAMHS mandatory
Hypoglycaemia	Nursing — monitoring	Safeguarding always considered
Collapse	Paediatrics if <18	

NEVER discharge if: No monitoring plan · No MDT agreement · Ongoing metabolic risk

SBAR · Must-Say · Fail Language

SBAR Escalation:
S: Eating disorder + instability · B: Vitals + ECG + labs · A: MEED positive/collapse risk · R: Urgent medical admission

✗ Fail Language	✓ Pass Language
"They seem okay for discharge"	"They meet admission criteria."
"Psychiatry can assess first"	"Medical stabilisation FIRST."
"Let's explore psychological causes first"	"Physical safety is the priority."
"They feel fine"	"They may feel fine but are medically unstable."

THINK — Complete Mnemonic Summary

Mnemonic	Purpose	Meaning
13-40-90	Core admission red flags	BMI <13 · HR <40 · SBP <90 or postural drop >20
MEED	Emergency admission check	Muscle (SUSS) · ECG · Electrolytes · Degree weight loss
SUSS	Functional frailty test	Sit up · Squat · Stand without arms — cardiac muscle proxy
START SLOW	Refeeding prevention	Thiamine first · Check electrolytes · Replace · Team · Slow advance · Ongoing phosphate
SBAR	Escalation	Situation · Background · Assessment · Recommendation

Final Exam Mantra

MEED = ADMIT · 13-40-90 = COLLAPSE · QTc + phosphate = survival · Glucose <3 = trolley · Refeeding = slow + thiamine · Uncertainty = admit

Gold Closing Statement:
"This is a patient with an eating disorder and significant medical instability. Based on their vital signs, ECG, and blood results, they meet criteria for urgent medical admission. They require medical ward admission with slow refeeding, thiamine before nutrition, and close electrolyte monitoring to prevent refeeding syndrome. I have escalated to the medical registrar via SBAR and involved the MDT including dietetics and psychiatry. The priority is medical stabilisation before psychiatric transfer."

13-40-90 admission red flags	MEED = admit any one trigger	QTc >450/460 ECG emergency	Phosphate <0.8 refeeding risk	Thiamine first before any feeding
SUSS test fail cardiac/muscle depletion	Glucose <3 = trolley no walking	Medical first psychiatry second	Paeds + centiles under-18 rule	SBAR mandatory every case

TOP 5 EXAMINER Q&A · EATING DISORDERS & ACUTE MEDICAL RISK	
Q1. Which findings mandate same-day medical assessment?	Use MEED red flags: BMI under 13, rapid weight loss, bradycardia under 40, hypotension, QTc prolongation, hypoglycaemia, hypokalaemia.
Q2. What is refeeding syndrome and who is at risk?	Dangerous fluid-electrolyte shifts (falling phosphate, potassium, magnesium) on refeeding after starvation: start low, monitor bloods daily, give thiamine.
Q3. Why check an ECG in anorexia?	Bradycardia and QTc prolongation predict arrhythmic death: an abnormal ECG changes the admission decision.
Q4. How do you weigh the conversation itself?	Non-judgemental, validate distress, avoid numbers battles, and never negotiate on safety.
Q5. Can treatment ever be compulsory?	Yes: under the MHA, feeding can be treatment for anorexia when life is at risk; senior and specialist decision.
CURVEBALL	Normal BMI but vomiting daily with potassium 2.8. Severity is not weight: this is a medical emergency: cardiac monitoring, replacement, and same-day specialist involvement.

CHAPTER 39 · HAEMATOLOGY & ONCOLOGY EMERGENCIES

Neutropenic Sepsis · Sickle Crisis · Transfusion Reaction · SVC Obstruction · Cord Compression · TLS · Hypercalcaemia

SICKLE · HOT · SVC · CORD · TUMOUR · TRALI vs TACO · SBAR

VERY HIGH · RED PATH · CAUTION — CRITICAL INSTANT FAIL RISK

Abbreviations used in this chapter: **ANC** Absolute Neutrophil Count · **JVP** Jugular Venous Pressure · **SVC** Superior Vena Cava · **TLS** Tumour Lysis Syndrome · **TRALI** Transfusion-Related Acute Lung Injury

Core Exam Focus: Starts treatment BEFORE diagnosis confirmation · Escalates early · Knows when NOT to delay

Examiner Lens: "Does this candidate recognise time-critical emergencies, initiate treatment without waiting for confirmation, and escalate appropriately?"

First Question in ANY Oncology Station: "Is this sepsis, spinal cord compression, airway compromise, or a transfusion reaction?"

Quick Reference — Critical Actions

Emergency	Critical Action
Neutropenic sepsis	IV antibiotics within 1 HOUR — do NOT wait for ANC
Cord compression	Dexamethasone IMMEDIATELY (high-dose, as per local protocol) + urgent MRI whole spine
Transfusion reaction	STOP transfusion immediately — save pack — call lab
Sickle crisis	Analgesia within 30 MINUTES — avoid meperidine
SVC obstruction	Sit upright + steroids + lower limb IVs only
TRALI vs TACO	Hypotensive = TRALI (fluids) · Hypertensive = TACO (furosemide)
Tumour lysis syndrome	IV fluids + allopurinol — avoid calcium unless symptomatic
Hypercalcaemia	IV fluids + bisphosphonates — avoid loop diuretics unless overloaded

Instant Fail

No antibiotics within 1h in neutropenic sepsis · Waits for ANC → fatal delay · Continues transfusion during reaction

Confuses TRALI vs TACO · Delays MRI in cord compression · Withholds steroids in cord compression

Misses stridor in SVC obstruction · Uses pethidine in sickle crisis · Gives O_2 routinely in sickle crisis

SAY — Golden Minute Script:
"This patient has a potential oncological emergency. My first question is: is this sepsis, spinal cord compression, airway compromise, or a transfusion reaction? I will assess ABCDE, identify the specific presentation, and initiate immediate treatment. For neutropenic sepsis — Sepsis Six and antibiotics within 1 hour. For transfusion reaction — STOP the transfusion and call the transfusion lab. For cord compression — urgent MRI and steroids with spinal precautions. I will involve haematology and oncology early."

Neutropenic Sepsis — Sepsis Six within 1 Hour

CAUTION — Post-chemo + fever = neutropenic sepsis until proven otherwise — do NOT wait for ANC result.

#	Sepsis Six — All within 1 Hour	Critical Point
1	Oxygen	Target SpO_2 94–98%
2	Blood cultures	Before antibiotics if possible — but do NOT delay
3	Broad-spectrum IV antibiotics	WITHIN 1 HOUR — most important step
4	IV fluids	If hypotensive
5	Lactate	Elevated = severe sepsis
6	Urine output monitoring	Aim >0.5 mL/kg/hour

Source control: Examine line sites · Skin + mouth · Perianal area: INSPECT ONLY (no rectal exam — bacteraemia risk). Line sepsis: if central line is the suspected source and patient is haemodynamically stable — remove line AFTER blood cultures, BEFORE antibiotics if possible. Do not delay antibiotics for an unstable patient.
SAY — Must-Say: "Post-chemo plus fever equals neutropenic sepsis until proven otherwise. Antibiotics within 1 hour — I will not wait for the FBC."

Sickle Cell Crisis — SICKLE Mnemonic

	SICKLE	Detail
S	Severe pain (vaso-occlusive)	Analgesia within 30 min — AVOID MEPERIDINE
I	Infection risk (asplenia)	Treat aggressively if fever
C	Chest syndrome (leading cause of death)	Dropping sats + chest pain + fever → CXR + haematology
K	Kidney (papillary necrosis)	U&E + urine
L	Leg ulcers	Wound review
E	Erection/priapism (>4h)	Exchange transfusion urgently

Management: ABCDE · Oxygen ONLY if SpO_2 <94% · IV fluids · Analgesia within 30 min (WHO ladder) · AVOID MEPERIDINE (seizures)

Exchange Transfusion Indications: Acute chest syndrome · Stroke · Priapism >4h · Multi-organ failure · Severe crisis not responding

SAY — Must-Say: "Analgesia within 30 minutes. I will avoid meperidine — it can cause seizures."

Transfusion Reactions — HOT + TRALI vs TACO

CAUTION — Any deterioration during transfusion = STOP transfusion immediately.

HOT: H — Haemolytic (ABO incompatibility) · O — Other: febrile/allergic · T — TRALI / TACO

Step	STOP Protocol
1	STOP transfusion immediately — keep line patent
2	ABCDE · oxygen · monitoring
3	Verify identity — check pack against patient — DO NOT discard pack — send to lab
4	IV fluids if hypotensive
5	Treat symptoms: antihistamines (allergic) · paracetamol (fever)
6	Call haematology + transfusion laboratory urgently
7	Investigations: FBC, U&E, cultures, repeat cross-match, direct Coombs test
8–9	Do NOT restart without haematology approval · Document time, reaction, actions

Feature	TACO — Fluid Overload	TRALI — Lung Injury
Blood pressure	Hypertensive	Hypotensive
Temperature	Normal	Febrile
JVP	Elevated	Normal or low
Treatment	Sit up + FUROSEMIDE	Fluids + ICU support

SVC Obstruction · Cord Compression

SVC Signs (SVC mnemonic): Swelling (face/neck/arms) · Veins distended · Cough + dyspnoea + Collateral circulation

Pemberton's sign: Raise both arms → face goes red or stridor develops = positive

SVC Actions: Sit upright (NEVER flat) · Lower limb IVs ONLY · Steroids · Stridor = call anaesthetics

Avoid: Sedation · supine position · upper limb IVs · DIURETICS (mechanical problem)

Cord Compression (CORD mnemonic):

C — Cancer history · O — Onset back pain (thoracic) · R — Radicular pain · D — Disability: leg weakness + sensory level + urinary retention + saddle anaesthesia

Cord Actions: STEROIDS IMMEDIATELY (no delay) · Urgent MRI whole spine (hours not days) · Log-roll flat · PR exam + saddle sensation · Catheterise if retention · Oncology + neurosurgery

SAY — Must-Say: "Steroids NOW — do NOT wait for MRI. Every hour counts to prevent paralysis."

Tumour Lysis Syndrome · Hypercalcaemia

Condition	Key Actions	Traps
Tumour Lysis Syndrome	IV fluids (first) · Allopurinol · Monitor $K^+/PO_4/Ca^{2+}$/urate · Rasburicase if established (check G6PD)	Do NOT give calcium unless symptomatic — precipitates with PO_4 → worsens renal failure
Hypercalcaemia	IV fluids (first) · Bisphosphonates (e.g. zoledronic acid) · Monitor Ca + renal function · Oncology review	Avoid loop diuretics UNLESS fluid overloaded

Stones, bones, groans, moans: Renal stones · bone pain · abdominal pain · confusion — symptoms of hypercalcaemia

Examiner Checklist

Neutropenic Sepsis ✓	Sickle Crisis ✓	Transfusion / Other ✓
First question asked	Analgesia within 30 min	STOPPED transfusion
Sepsis Six within 1 hour	Meperidine avoided	Pack saved + lab called
Antibiotics — did NOT wait for ANC	Oxygen only if SpO_2 <94%	TRALI vs TACO distinguished
No rectal exam	Acute chest syndrome monitored	SVC: sat up + lower limb IVs
Haematology + ICU involved	Exchange indications known	Cord: steroids + MRI + PR exam

Final Exam Mantra

FIRST QUESTION: Sepsis? Cord? Airway? Transfusion reaction?

N — Neutropenic: Sepsis Six + antibiotics within 1 HOUR — no rectal exam — do NOT wait for ANC

S — Sickle: Analgesia within 30 min — AVOID MEPERIDINE — oxygen only if SpO_2 <94%

C — Cord: Steroids IMMEDIATELY + urgent MRI (hours not days) + log-roll flat

T — Transfusion: STOP + save pack + call lab + TRALI vs TACO

C — SVC: Sit up + lower limb IVs + Pemberton's sign + NO diuretics

T — TLS: IV fluids + allopurinol — NO calcium unless symptomatic

H — Hypercalcaemia: IV fluids + bisphosphonates — NO loop diuretics unless overloaded

TRALI = hypotensive + febrile → fluids + ICU · TACO = hypertensive → furosemide

Abx within 1 hour neutropenic sepsis	No ANC wait fatal delay	No rectal exam bacteraemia risk	Analgesia 30 min sickle crisis	Avoid meperidine seizure risk
STOP transfusion immediately always	TACO = furosemide hypertensive	TRALI = fluids+ICU hypotensive + fever	Dexamethasone now cord compression	No upper limb IVs SVC obstruction

TOP 5 EXAMINER Q&A · HAEMATOLOGY & ONCOLOGY EMERGENCIES	
Q1. Define neutropenic sepsis and the time target.	Neutrophils below 0.5 with fever or sepsis signs after chemotherapy: broad-spectrum antibiotics within one hour, before results.
Q2. Back pain in a cancer patient: what must you exclude?	Metastatic spinal cord compression: neurological examination, urgent whole-spine MRI, dexamethasone while arranging it.
Q3. Acute chest pain in sickle cell disease?	Acute chest syndrome: oxygen, analgesia within 30 minutes, fluids, senior and haematology involvement early.
Q4. Fever during a blood transfusion: first actions?	Stop the transfusion, reassess the patient, check identity and the unit, and escalate per transfusion protocol.
Q5. What suggests tumour lysis syndrome?	High potassium, phosphate and urate with low calcium and AKI after starting treatment: fluids and urgent senior input.
CURVEBALL	A chemotherapy patient "just feels off" with a normal temperature. Neutropenic sepsis can be afebrile: assess fully and treat on suspicion: the hour rule still applies.

CHAPTER 40 · ACUTE SURGICAL EMERGENCIES

Septic Arthritis · Compartment Syndrome · Anastomotic Leak · Post-Op Fever

HUT JOINT · CAST OFF · LEAK FIRST · 5 Ws+1

VERY HIGH · ED / Acute Surgical Take / Post-Op Ward · CAUTION — INSTANT FAIL RISK

Abbreviations used in this chapter: **COPD** Chronic Obstructive Pulmonary Disease · **CTPA** CT Pulmonary Angiogram · **DVT** Deep Vein Thrombosis · **NBM** Nil By Mouth · **NEWS2** National Early Warning Score 2 · **PE** Pulmonary Embolism · **USS** Ultrasound Scan

Core Focus: Recognise early, act without delay, verbalise "what I am NOT doing", reassess every 15 minutes

Emergency	Critical Action
Septic arthritis	Unable to weight-bear = KEY sign · IV antibiotics within 1 hour · NEVER inject LA · ask pregnancy
Compartment syndrome	Do NOT wait for pulses · Remove cast NOW · Reassess every 15 minutes
Anastomotic leak	Unexplained tachycardia = earliest sign · Do NOT wait for fever · Do NOT use D-dimer
Post-op fever	5 Ws+1: Wind (D1-2) · Water (D3-5) · Wound (D5-7) · Walk (D5-7) · Wonder (any) · +1 Drain/line

Instant Fail (INSTANT-FAIL BEHAVIOURS)

Septic Arthritis	Compartment Syndrome	Anastomotic Leak
Delayed antibiotics (aspirate first)	Waiting for loss of pulses	Waiting for fever before escalation
Injecting LA into joint	Elevating limb above heart	Using D-dimer post-op
Missing "unable to weight-bear"	Single neurovascular check only	Attributing tachycardia to pain
No pregnancy check (female)	Failure to document neurovascular	Ignoring rising NEWS2 or lactate

Station Recognition · Golden Minute Scripts

Presentation	Think → Golden Minute Script
Hot joint + unable to weight-bear	HUT JOINT → "Not injecting LA, not waiting for imaging. IV abx within 1 hour. Ortho informed. Pregnancy asked."
Pain out of proportion + worse on passive stretch	CAST OFF → "Removing cast now — limb at heart level. NOT elevated. Reassessing q15min."
Post-op day 3 + unexplained tachycardia	LEAK FIRST → "NOT waiting for fever. NOT using D-dimer. Senior NOW. CT after senior review."

Presentation	Think → Golden Minute Script
Post-op fever any day	5 Ws+1 → Day-based differential. Remove catheter/lines if indicated.
Elderly + delirium only	Surgical emergency until proven → NEWS2 trend + lactate — no fever does NOT exclude

THINK — Core Mnemonics — HUT JOINT · CAST OFF · LEAK FIRST

	HUT JOINT	CAST OFF	LEAK FIRST
1	Hot joint	Cast removal NOW	Lactate rising
2	Unable to weight-bear	Analgesia + reassess	Elderly no fever
3	Tachycardia	Stretch pain (diagnostic)	Abdominal pain
4	Joint aspirate	Tension	Know tachy = earliest
5	Ortho referral	Ortho referral	Fever? Do NOT wait
6	IV abx <1hr	Fasciotomy	Investigations: CT after senior
7	Never inject LA	Frequent reassess q15min	Return to theatre
8	Time-critical · ask pregnancy		Senior NOW · Trend matters

Surgical ABCDE — Verbalise Each Step

	Key Actions	Verbalise
A	Airway patent	"Airway patent and protected."
B	SpO_2 <94% → O_2 (88–92% if COPD)	"SpO_2 92% — giving oxygen now."
C	HR (earliest sign) · BP (late) · Lactate · Urine output · IV fluids · NEWS2 trend	"HR 112 — tachycardia is my earliest warning sign. NEWS2 trend rising — escalating now."
D	Pain score · Glucose · Drug chart	"Pain score 8/10 — checking drug chart."
E	Remove dressings · Inspect wound	"Elderly may not mount fever — relying on NEWS2 trend."

Reassessment: Unstable = every 15 min · Deteriorating = immediately · ALWAYS document neurovascular status

Post-Op Fever — 5 Ws+1

W	Timing	Cause	Action
Wind	Day 1–2	Atelectasis	Incentive spirometry · mobilise · CXR
Water	Day 3–5	UTI	Urine dipstick · remove catheter
Wound	Day 5–7	Surgical site infection	Inspect · swab · antibiotics
Walk	Day 5–7	DVT/PE	Duplex USS or CTPA
Wonder	Any time	Drug fever / transfusion reaction	Review drug chart
+1	Any time	Drain or line infection	Inspect site · remove if infected

Special Populations · SBAR Escalation

Elderly: Delirium as ONLY sign · No fever · Subtle tachycardia → Escalate early — do NOT wait for fever — trend NEWS2 + lactate
Child: Pseudoparalysis, refuses to walk → Septic arthritis until proven — involve paediatrics
Immunocompromised: No fever · Slow CRP rise → Escalate · Adjust antibiotics

SBAR Escalation:
S: "Time-critical surgical emergency — [HUT JOINT / CAST OFF / LEAK FIRST]."
B: "[Age], post-op day [X]. NEWS2 rising. Key finding: [unable to weight-bear / passive stretch pain / unexplained tachycardia]."
A: "ABCDE done. Concern: [septic arthritis / compartment syndrome / anastomotic leak]."
R: "Need review within minutes. May need [washout / fasciotomy / return to theatre]."
CAUTION — If senior unreachable: Call again · Switchboard · If deteriorating → call 2222

Examiner Checklist

Septic Arthritis ✓	Compartment Syndrome ✓	Anastomotic Leak ✓
"Unable to weight-bear" identified	Cast removed immediately	Tachycardia identified as earliest sign
Pregnancy asked (female)	Limb at heart level (NOT elevated)	Fever NOT waited for
Blood cultures taken	Pain on passive stretch identified	D-dimer NOT used
Joint aspirated	Pulselessness = LATE sign stated	Lactate checked + trend documented
IV abx within 1 hour	Neurovascular status documented	CT arranged AFTER senior review
LA NOT injected	Ortho referred · fasciotomy considered	NBM + IV fluids + IV abx started

Final Exam Mantra

HUT JOINT: Hot · Unable to weight-bear (KEY) · Tachy · Joint aspirate · Ortho · IV abx <1hr · Never inject LA · Time-critical

CAST OFF: Cast removal NOW · Analgesia+reassess · Stretch pain (diagnostic) · Tension · Ortho · Fasciotomy · Frequent reassess q15min

LEAK FIRST: Lactate rising · Elderly no fever · Abdominal pain · Know tachy = earliest · Fever? Do NOT wait · CT after senior · Return to theatre · Senior NOW

5 Ws+1: Wind (D1-2) · Water (D3-5) · Wound (D5-7) · Walk (D5-7) · Wonder (any) · +1 Drain/line

NEVER: D-dimer · Wait for fever in elderly · Wait for pulses · Inject LA · Elevate compartment limb

Unable to weight-bear septic arthritis KEY sign	LA = instant fail never inject joint	Abx within 1 hour before aspirate results	Remove cast NOW compartment syndrome	Pulses = late sign don't wait
Reassess q15min every time document	Tachycardia = earliest anastomotic leak	No D-dimer post-op always raised	No fever in elderly trend NEWS2 + lactate	Senior NOW before CT

TOP 5 EXAMINER Q&A · ACUTE SURGICAL EMERGENCIES	
Q1. Hot swollen joint: what must happen before antibiotics?	Joint aspiration for urgent Gram stain and culture: septic arthritis destroys cartilage within days.
Q2. Pain out of proportion in a casted limb?	Compartment syndrome: split the cast, elevate to heart level, urgent orthopaedic review for fasciotomy: do not wait for pulselessness.
Q3. Day-5 post-laparotomy fever and tachycardia?	Think anastomotic leak: examine the abdomen, septic screen, escalate to the surgical team urgently.
Q4. Framework for post-operative fever?	The 5 Ws by timing: wind, water, wound, walking (VTE), wonder drugs: plus the anastomosis after bowel surgery.
Q5. When is an urgent CT abdomen justified over observation?	Peritonism, sepsis without source, or suspected leak: but an unstable patient goes to theatre, not the scanner.
CURVEBALL	The orthopaedic registrar says "observe overnight" but compartment pressures are rising clinically. Re-escalate: state findings, time-critical risk, and request consultant review: polite persistence saves the limb.

CHAPTER 41 · CHRONIC PAIN & PERSISTENT PHYSICAL SYMPTOMS

RED FLAGS · BATHE · Biopsychosocial · Pacing · Yellow Flags · Fit Note · DVLA

VERY HIGH · GP / Outpatient / Pain Clinic · CAUTION — MODERATE INSTANT FAIL RISK

Abbreviations used in this chapter: **CBT** Cognitive Behavioural Therapy · **DVLA** Driver & Vehicle Licensing Agency

Examiner Lens: "Will this doctor recognise chronic pain safely, validate the patient, avoid dismissing symptoms, and create a realistic biopsychosocial plan without over-investigating?"

Golden Rule: "First question: Are there any NEW or CHANGING red flags needing investigation — or is this persistent symptoms with previous reassuring tests?"

Strong Candidate: Screens red flags first · Says "Your symptoms are real" · Validates impact · Uses BATHE · Explores yellow flags · Biopsychosocial formulation · Avoids over-investigation

Instant Fail

Skips red flag screening · Says "It's just stress" · Uses "psychosomatic" or "all in your head"

Dismisses because tests are normal · Over-investigates without new red flags · Prescribes opioids casually

Generic advice ("just exercise more") · Ignores psychosocial factors · No safety-netting

Sick note without functional assessment · Says "There's nothing more we can do"

Station Recognition · Golden Opening

If you hear...	Think...
"Nobody can find what's wrong."	Persistent physical symptoms
"I need another scan."	Expectation management
"You don't believe me."	Therapeutic alliance at risk
"I can't work because of pain."	Functional assessment / fit note
Fibromyalgia / IBS / CFS review	Functional syndrome management

SAY — Golden Opening Script:

"Thank you for telling me about this. I can hear how difficult this has been. First, I'd like to check for any new red flags that need investigation, then understand how this is affecting your life so we can make a plan together. Is that okay?"

8-Minute OSCE Flow

0–1 min	Introduce · agenda · invite story
1–3 min	Listen + validate impact
3–4 min	Screen RED FLAGS — first priority

4–5 min	Explore YELLOW FLAGS
5–6 min	Build biopsychosocial explanation
6–7 min	Management plan + pacing
7–8 min	Safety-net + referrals + follow-up

Red Flags — Organic Disease Screen

	RED FLAGS	When to Re-Investigate
R	Recent / new symptoms	New symptoms
E	Escalating severity	Change in pattern
D	Drama: fever, weight loss, night sweats	New neurological findings
F	Function loss sudden	Systemic features
L	Localising neurological signs	Failure to improve unexpectedly
A	Age >50 or <20	
G	Gait / balance change	
S	Systemic symptoms	

SAY — Must-Say: "I investigate when the clinical picture changes — not simply to repeat previous normal tests."

Yellow Flags · BATHE Validation

Yellow Flag	Why It Matters
Fear of movement	Leads to avoidance and deconditioning
Anxiety / low mood	Amplifies pain perception
Catastrophising	Increases disability
Passive coping	Reduces rehabilitation engagement
Work stress	Delays recovery
Social isolation	Worsens function
Overprotective family	Reinforces illness behaviour

Mental Health Screen: "Has the pain ever felt so overwhelming that you've felt hopeless or thought about harming yourself?"
CAUTION — If YES → urgent mental health assessment.

	BATHE Validation Framework
B	"How has this been affecting your life?"

	BATHE Validation Framework
A	"How does that make you feel?"
T	"What troubles you most?"
H	"How are you coping with that?"
E	"That sounds incredibly difficult." (Empathy statement)

Double Validation:
Symptom: "Your pain is real." · Impact: "I can see how much this is affecting your sleep and daily life."

Biopsychosocial Formulation · Safe Language

Domain	Explore / Script
Biological	"How is your sleep and energy?"
Psychological	"How has this affected your mood?"
Social	"How is this affecting work and life at home?"

Formulation Script: "Your symptoms are real, but they're also affecting your sleep, mood, and confidence with activity. Because you're worried about making things worse, you've become less active — and that can keep the cycle going. That's something we can work on together."

Smoke Alarm Analogy: "Think of the nervous system like a smoke alarm that has become too sensitive — going off too easily. The alarm is real, but it doesn't always mean damage is happening. We can help calm and retrain the system."

✗ Avoid	✓ Say Instead
"MUS"	"Persistent physical symptoms"
"Psychosomatic"	"Symptoms affected by the nervous system"
"It's psychological."	"Stress and physical symptoms can affect each other."
"Nothing is wrong."	"The tests are reassuring, which is good news."
"It's all in your head."	"Your symptoms are real."
"Just exercise more."	"We'll build activity gradually and safely."

Management Plan · Pacing · Medication Safety

Step	Action
Education	Explain persistent pain safely — smoke alarm analogy
Activity: Pacing	Graded activity — avoid boom-bust
Sleep	Sleep hygiene
Mood	Address anxiety/depression

Step	Action
Medication review	Reduce opioids/gabapentinoids if appropriate
Referral	Physio · Pain clinic · Psychology/CBT · Social prescribing
Follow-up	Review progress regularly

Pacing — Boom-Bust Cycle: Good day → overactivity → flare/crash → prolonged recovery. Aim for steady sustainable activity instead.

SAY — Must-Say: "Many people do too much on good days and then crash. Instead, we aim for a steady, sustainable level of activity."

Opioid Safety: "Long-term opioids often become less effective and can sometimes worsen chronic pain. We'd reduce gradually with support rather than stopping suddenly."

Fit Note · DVLA · Safety-Netting

Fit Note — Golden Rule: Assess FUNCTION — not diagnosis.

"Tell me how your symptoms affect your ability to work." · "Could adjusted duties or reduced hours help you stay connected to work safely?"

DVLA Advice: Patients must NOT drive if: pain impairs safe control · medication causes drowsiness · concentration is impaired.

SAY — Must-Say: "If your medication or symptoms affect alertness or safe control of the vehicle, you must not drive."

Safety-Netting:

Return for: new neurological symptoms · fever / weight loss / night sweats · worsening function · mental health deterioration (same-day)

Examiner Checklist

✓ Red flags screened FIRST · ✓ Symptoms validated · ✓ BATHE structure used

✓ Yellow flags explored · ✓ Biopsychosocial formulation built · ✓ Avoided dismissive language

✓ Avoided unnecessary investigations · ✓ Explained pacing · ✓ Medication risks discussed

✓ Appropriate referrals offered · ✓ Fit note assessed functionally · ✓ Driving advice given

✓ Safety-netting provided · ✓ Follow-up arranged

Final Exam Mantra

RED FLAGS first · Validate symptom AND impact · Use BATHE · Explore yellow flags · Build biopsychosocial formulation

Say "persistent physical symptoms" · Avoid over-investigation · Use smoke alarm analogy · Focus on pacing and function

Assess function for fit notes · Sedating meds = driving advice · Always safety-net and follow up

Gold Closing Statement:

"Your symptoms are real, and I can see how much they're affecting your life. We've screened for red flags and found nothing suggesting a dangerous cause, which is reassuring. Several factors — sleep, stress, reduced activity, and nervous system over-sensitivity — are contributing together. Rather than repeating more tests, we'll focus on function and quality of life through pacing, gradual activity, and specialist support. I'd like to review you in a few weeks. If symptoms change or new red flags appear, please seek review sooner."

RED FLAGS first before any reassurance	"Your pain is real" validate always	BATHE framework B-A-T-H-E	Yellow flags maintain chronicity	Biopsychosocial 3-domain formulation
Smoke alarm analogy sensitised nervous system	Pacing not boom-bust sustainable activity	No over-investigation no new red flags rule	Fit note = function not diagnosis	DVLA if sedating meds driving safety

TOP 5 EXAMINER Q&A · CHRONIC PAIN & PERSISTENT PHYSICAL SYMPTOMS	
Q1. How do you explain chronic primary pain without dismissing it?	The pain is real: the alarm system itself has become sensitised; investigations exclude damage but do not measure pain.
Q2. What are yellow flags?	Psychosocial barriers to recovery: fear-avoidance, low mood, catastrophising, work issues: they predict chronicity.
Q3. Why is pacing central to management?	Boom-and-bust cycles worsen disability; planned, graded consistent activity rebuilds function.
Q4. What is the role of opioids in chronic primary pain?	Minimal: poor long-term evidence and significant harm; avoid initiation and plan reduction where already prescribed.
Q5. How do you handle the fit note conversation?	Focus on what they can do: amended duties and phased return keep people connected to work, which improves outcomes.
CURVEBALL	"So you're saying it's all in my head?" Address it directly: the pain is absolutely real and physical: it is the processing, not imagination: validation is the treatment's foundation.

CHAPTER 42 · EARLY PREGNANCY BLEEDING & ECTOPIC PREGNANCY

BLEED · ECTOPIC · SHARP · 1-4-7-W · LOSS · SPIKES · Anti-D

CORE · ED / EPAU / GP Urgent · CAUTION — HIGH INSTANT FAIL RISK

Abbreviations used in this chapter: **ERPC** Evacuation of Retained Products of Conception · **IUP** Intrauterine Pregnancy · **TVUSS** Transvaginal Ultrasound Scan · **USS** Ultrasound Scan

Instant Fail Reasoning Cards

Cognitive Error	Instant-Fail Behaviour	Saving Rule
Accepting the history — contraception, a recent period, "not sexually active" — as sufficient to exclude pregnancy.	Not performing a pregnancy test in a woman of reproductive age presenting with abdominal pain or vaginal bleeding.	Test every woman of reproductive age with abdominal pain or vaginal bleeding, whatever the history offered. "I'd like to do a pregnancy test. We do this for everyone with these symptoms — it isn't about anything you've told me."
Deciding it is not an ectopic because the picture does not fit — the pain sounds musculoskeletal or gastrointestinal, or the patient has none of the classic risk factors.	Accepting a non-gynaecological explanation for lower abdominal pain, or dismissing ectopic for want of risk factors, before a pregnancy test is done.	Ectopic stays in the differential until a pregnancy test says otherwise — whatever the pain sounds like, whatever the risk profile. "I know the pain doesn't sound gynaecological, and you don't have the usual risk factors. But the way we exclude an ectopic pregnancy is a pregnancy test — so I'm going to do that before we go any further."
Treating investigation as the next step in a patient who has already declared herself unstable.	Performing or awaiting ultrasound or serum β-hCG in a haemodynamically unstable woman with suspected ectopic, rather than referring immediately.	Unstable, positive pregnancy test and abdominal pain is a ruptured ectopic until proven otherwise — refer for urgent surgical assessment without waiting for imaging. "You're unstable, and with a positive pregnancy test and abdominal pain this could be an ectopic pregnancy. I'm not waiting for a scan — I'm referring you to the surgical team now for an urgent assessment."

THINK — Core Truth: All early pregnancy pain + bleeding = ectopic until proven otherwise.
First Question (MUST SAY): "First I need to check if you are stable and rule out an ectopic pregnancy."
Examiner focus: "Can you NOT miss ectopic, stabilise first, interpret hCG/USS correctly, and break bad news safely?"

Stable vs Unstable — Critical Split

UNSTABLE = Surgical Emergency	STABLE = Structured Assessment
Hypotension / collapse	Proceed to history + investigations
Tachycardia	BLEED mnemonic
Shoulder tip pain	TVUSS safe to proceed
Peritonism / rigid abdomen	Serial β-hCG possible
Syncope	Methotrexate/expectant options

UNSTABLE Action (no delay, no scan):
✓ 2 large-bore cannulas · ✓ IV fluids · ✓ Oxygen · ✓ Cross-match · ✓ Analgesia · ✓ Call gynae registrar NOW · ✓ Prep theatre
✗ NEVER send unstable patient for ultrasound.

SHARP Rupture Signs · Investigations

	SHARP	Action
S	Shoulder pain	Blood under diaphragm → immediate surgery
H	Hypotension	Haemorrhagic shock → resuscitate + surgical
A	Adrenaline signs (tachycardia)	Compensatory shock → cross-match + theatre
R	Rigid abdomen	Peritonism → haemoperitoneum
P	Peritonism	Generalised tenderness → laparotomy

SAY — Must-Say: "Any ONE of SHARP = immediate surgical emergency — do NOT send for scan."

Step	Investigation	Purpose
1	Urine pregnancy test	Confirm pregnancy FIRST
2	Serum β-hCG (serial)	Trend guides diagnosis
3	TVUSS	Gold standard — IUP? Empty uterus? Mass?
4	Blood group + rhesus	Anti-D if indicated — check EARLY
5	FBC	Baseline Hb
6	Group & save / cross-match	If significant bleeding or unstable

β-hCG Interpretation · Core Diagnoses

β-hCG Pattern	Meaning	Action
Rise ≥63% in 48h	Likely viable IUP	USS to confirm

β-hCG Pattern	Meaning	Action
Plateau or slow rise	Ectopic until proven otherwise	Treat as ectopic — serial USS
Falling	Miscarriage / resolving PUL	Monitor until negative

Discriminatory Zone: β-hCG >1500 + empty uterus = ectopic until proven otherwise — do NOT reassure.
PUL Warning: "PUL is not a diagnosis — it is a risk state until ectopic is excluded. Do NOT reassure."

Diagnosis	Key Feature
Threatened miscarriage	Closed os · IUP + fetal heartbeat — most continue
Inevitable miscarriage	Open os · products visible
Incomplete miscarriage	Open os · retained products
Missed miscarriage	Closed os · sac present · no heartbeat
Ectopic	Empty uterus + adnexal mass · constant unilateral pain
Septic miscarriage	Fever + foul discharge + tachycardia
PUL	Positive test · nothing on scan — risk state (NOT a diagnosis)

Management Options · Methotrexate · Anti-D

Offer ALL Three — Shared Decision:
Expectant: Natural, unpredictable, may take weeks · Medical (methotrexate): Avoids surgery, but rupture still possible in first week · Surgical: Definitive
SAY — Must-Say: "Let's decide together which option suits you best — what matters most to you?"

Methotrexate ✓ Eligible	✗ Contraindicated	1-4-7-W Schedule
Stable	Unstable / ruptured	Day 1: Single IM dose
Unruptured	Cannot follow up	Day 4: Check β-hCG (may rise — do NOT worry)
No fetal heartbeat	Breastfeeding	Day 7: Must fall from Day 4
β-hCG typically <5000	Liver disease	Weekly: Until negative
Mass <35mm	Immunodeficiency	

CAUTION — Critical Warnings:
"Rupture can still occur in the first week — severe pain or shoulder tip pain → A&E immediately."
Avoid breastfeeding ≥12 weeks · Pregnancy 3 months · NSAIDs / alcohol / folate

SAY — Anti-D (Exam Favourite) — Give within 72h if Rh-negative:

<12 weeks YES: ERPC · Ectopic · Molar · Significant/recurrent bleeding

<12 weeks NOT routinely: Complete miscarriage (no intervention) · Threatened miscarriage (minimal bleeding)

>12 weeks: ANY miscarriage or bleeding event → YES

SAY — Must-Say: "Because you are rhesus negative, we need to give you anti-D within 72 hours to protect future pregnancies."

Breaking Bad News — LOSS + SPIKES

ALWAYS SAY: "This is not your fault. Nothing you did caused this."

LOSS Framework	SPIKES (Short Version)
L — Listen (allow silence, do NOT rush)	S — Setting: private room, sit
O — Offer empathy: "I am so sorry."	P — Perception: "What do you understand?"
S — Share: "The pregnancy has not continued."	I — Invitation: "May I explain?"
S — Support: options + written info + self-harm screen	K — Knowledge: "The pregnancy has not continued."
	E — Emotions: pause, allow tears
	S — Summary: next steps + support

Safety-Net — Mandatory Marks

Symptom	Action
Severe abdominal pain	A&E immediately
Shoulder tip pain	A&E immediately — rupture until proven
Dizziness / collapse	A&E immediately
Heavy bleeding (>1 pad/hour)	A&E immediately
Fever	A&E immediately

Post-Methotrexate: "Even though the injection is working, the tube can still rupture in the first week."

3-Week Rule: "Pregnancy test in 3 weeks — if still positive, you must return."

Safeguarding: "Do you feel safe at home? Any thoughts of harming yourself?"

Examiner Checklist · Mnemonic Summary

Assessment: ✓ Stability first · ✓ Bleeding quantified · ✓ Pregnancy confirmed · ✓ Rhesus checked · ✓ Safeguarding asked

Diagnosis: ✓ SHARP recognised · ✓ β-hCG trend interpreted · ✓ Discriminatory zone stated · ✓ PUL = risk state

Management: ✓ All 3 options offered · ✓ Methotrexate eligibility · ✓ 1-4-7-W explained · ✓ Rupture warning given

Communication: ✓ LOSS/SPIKES used · ✓ "Not your fault" said · ✓ Self-harm screen · ✓ Safety-net given

Mnemonic	Use	Meaning
BLEED	Early pregnancy bleeding	BP/stability · Location · Exclude ectopic · Explain options · D status (Anti-D 72h)
SHARP	Rupture red flags	Shoulder · Hypotension · Adrenaline signs · Rigid · Peritonism → immediate surgery
1-4-7-W	Methotrexate follow-up	Day 1 dose · Day 4 β-hCG · Day 7 must fall · Weekly until negative
LOSS	Breaking bad news	Listen · Offer empathy · Share information · Support + self-harm screen

Final Exam Mantra

FIRST: Stable or unstable? → Unstable = 2 cannulas + fluids + O_2 + morphine + cross-match + surgery — do NOT scan

β-hCG: Rise ≥63% = IUP · Plateau/slow = ectopic · Falling = miscarriage

Discriminatory Zone: >1500 + empty uterus = ectopic — do NOT reassure with PUL

SHARP: Shoulder · Hypotension · Adrenaline signs · Rigid · Peritonism → immediate surgery

Methotrexate: 1-4-7-W · Warn rupture first week · Avoid breastfeeding ≥12 weeks

Anti-D: <12w YES for ERPC/ectopic/molar/significant bleeding · NOT for minimal threatened

"This is not your fault." · "Do you feel safe at home?" · 3-week pregnancy test rule

Ectopic first unstable = no scan	SHARP = surgery any one sign	No scan if unstable theatre directly	β-hCG ≥63% rise viable IUP	Plateau = ectopic treat as ectopic
>1500 + empty discriminatory zone	1-4-7-W methotrexate schedule	Rupture first week warn always	Anti-D 72h Rh-negative rule	"Not your fault" mandatory phrase

TOP 5 EXAMINER Q&A · EARLY PREGNANCY BLEEDING & ECTOPIC PREGNANCY

Q1. Abdominal pain plus bleeding in early pregnancy: default assumption?	Ectopic pregnancy until location is confirmed: urgent EPAU referral or emergency admission if unstable.

TOP 5 EXAMINER Q&A · EARLY PREGNANCY BLEEDING & ECTOPIC PREGNANCY	
Q2. Shoulder-tip pain in this context means?	Diaphragmatic irritation from haemoperitoneum: a ruptured ectopic: resuscitate and call gynaecology immediately.
Q3. Who needs anti-D after bleeding?	Rhesus-negative women after surgical management or significant sensitising events per gestation-specific guidance.
Q4. Management options for confirmed miscarriage?	Expectant, medical or surgical: explain all three neutrally and support her choice.
Q5. How do you communicate pregnancy loss?	Plainly and compassionately: avoid “at least” phrases, acknowledge grief, offer follow-up and written information.
CURVEBALL	Her scan is “pregnancy of unknown location” and she wants to go home for the weekend. Safety-net hard: ectopic is not excluded: explicit return advice, serial hCG plan, and document her understanding.

CHAPTER 43 · O&G EMERGENCIES

Pre-Eclampsia · Eclampsia · PPH · Shoulder Dystocia · Cord Prolapse · Reduced Fetal Movements

P-PRESS · HELPERR · ELEVATE · KICK CHART · 4 Ts · RARO · 6× SBAR

CORE · GREEN PATH · CAUTION — HIGH INSTANT FAIL RISK

Abbreviations used in this chapter: **AFI** Amniotic Fluid Index · **BPP** Biophysical Profile · **CTG** Cardiotocography · **EBL** Estimated Blood Loss · **GDM** Gestational Diabetes Mellitus · **IUGR** Intrauterine Growth Restriction · **MHP** Major Haemorrhage Protocol · **NEWS2** National Early Warning Score 2 · **PE** Pulmonary Embolism · **PPH** Postpartum Haemorrhage · **RFM** Reduced Fetal Movements · **TXA** Tranexamic Acid · **USS** Ultrasound Scan

THINK — Core Rule: MOTHER FIRST → BABY SECOND → PROTOCOL ALWAYS. Wrong sequence = instant fail.

SAY — First Question (Every Station): "Is this mother or baby at immediate risk? MOTHER FIRST, BABY SECOND."

SAY — Golden Minute Script: "This is an obstetric emergency — I have identified [condition]. I am calling for help immediately. My priority is maternal safety first, then fetal rescue. I will initiate the protocol now and keep you informed throughout."

P-PRESS	Emergency	5-Second Recall Line
P	Pre-eclampsia	ABCDE → labetalol/nifedipine → $MgSO_4$ 4g load → RARO 24h → plan delivery
P	PPH	Massage → oxytocin → ergometrine → carboprost → misoprostol → TXA 1g → MHP
R	Reduced fetal movements	CTG first → USS → BPP → BPP ≤4 = deliver NOW
E	Eclampsia	Airway + lateral tilt → $MgSO_4$ NOW → call anaesthetics
S	Shoulder dystocia	HELPERR — NO fundal pressure — McRoberts → suprapubic → posterior arm → 5 min
S	Cord prolapse	ELEVATE — hand UP (do NOT remove) → knee-chest → tocolysis → cat-1 CS

Instant Fail Triggers

Trigger	Why It Fails
Fundal pressure (shoulder dystocia)	**Worsens impaction → brachial plexus injury — INSTANT FAIL RISK**
Removing hand (cord prolapse)	**Cord compression → fetal death — INSTANT FAIL RISK**
$MgSO_4$ without reflex check	Respiratory arrest from toxicity
Ergometrine in hypertension	Severe hypertensive crisis
Carboprost in asthma	Bronchospasm

Trigger	Why It Fails
Wrong uterotonic sequence	Oxytocin must be first
Stopping $MgSO_4$ too early	Postpartum eclampsia risk — continue 24h
No CTG for reduced movements	Missed fetal compromise — instant fail
BPP ≤4 not acted on	Every minute of delay matters
No escalation / works alone	Unsafe obstetric practice

1. Pre-Eclampsia · Eclampsia

Diagnosis: BP ≥160/110 + proteinuria = severe pre-eclampsia — treat within 1 hour.
Postpartum PE: Can occur UP TO 4 WEEKS after delivery — do NOT stop monitoring early.

Step	Action	Detail
1	ABCDE + lateral tilt	Prevents aortocaval compression
2	Call obstetrician + anaesthetics	Immediately
3	Labetalol 200mg PO / 20mg IV	OR Nifedipine 10mg PO → target <160/110
4	$MgSO_4$ 4g IV loading	Over 5–10 min → continue 24h after delivery / last seizure
5	RARO monitoring hourly	Reflexes + Airway/RR + Renal output + O_2/GCS — RARO monitoring MEOWS (Modified Early Obstetric Warning Score) = maternity equivalent of NEWS2. Any single red score OR MEOWS ≥2 = immediate senior review.
6	Fluid restriction	Prevent pulmonary oedema
7	Plan delivery	Gestation + stability + senior decision

RARO: R — Reflexes (loss → STOP) · A — Airway/RR (<12 → STOP) · R — Renal output · O — O_2/GCS
Antidote: Calcium gluconate 1g IV
Eclampsia: Airway → lateral tilt → $MgSO_4$ NOW → call anaesthetics → continuous monitoring

2. Postpartum Haemorrhage (PPH)

Trigger: Act on CLINICAL SUSPICION — do not wait for measured blood loss.
Primary PPH: Within 24h of delivery · Secondary PPH: 24h to 6 weeks postpartum
MHP: Activate if >1500 mL OR haemodynamic instability

4 Ts Causes: Tone (uterine atony) · Tissue (retained products) · Trauma (tears/rupture) · Thrombin (coagulopathy)

#	Uterotonics Sequence	Contraindication
1	Oxytocin 10 units IM/slow IV — ALWAYS FIRST (immediate bolus: Step 1). Then: oxytocin 40 IU infusion over 4h (maintenance: Step 2). These are two different steps — bolus then infusion. Never give 40 IU as a bolus.	None
2	Ergometrine 500 mcg IM	✗ Hypertension / pre-eclampsia
3	Carboprost 250 mcg IM	✗ Asthma
4	Misoprostol 800 mcg PR	None
+	Tranexamic acid 1g IV — within 3 hours	Non-negotiable

If medical fails: Bakri balloon → B-lynch suture → theatre (do NOT delay after 2 uterotonics fail)

3. Shoulder Dystocia — HELPERR

Trigger: Turtle sign after head delivery. Deliver within 5 minutes. Call NEONATOLOGY immediately.
NEVER fundal pressure — INSTANT FAIL RISK. Document time, manoeuvres, personnel, outcomes.

H	Help — neonatology	Call IMMEDIATELY
E	Episiotomy	Creates space
L	McRoberts (legs)	Hyperflex thighs onto abdomen
P	Pressure suprapubic ONLY	✗ NOT fundal — suprapubic only, above symphysis
E	Enter manoeuvres	Rubin II / Wood's screw
R	Remove posterior arm	Sweep arm across chest
R	Roll over (Gaskin)	All-fours manoeuvre

4. Cord Prolapse — ELEVATE

Trigger: Cord visible after ROM — IMMEDIATE delivery. Hand UP — DO NOT REMOVE until baby delivered.

E	Elevate (hand UP)	DO NOT REMOVE — removing hand = fetal death

L	Legs — knee-chest / Trendelenburg	Reduces cord compression
E	Expel — do NOT touch cord	Handling causes vasospasm
V	Veins — IV access + tocolysis	Terbutaline 0.25mg SC if contracting
A	Amniotic — keep membranes intact	If possible
T	Transfer — category-1 CS	Do NOT delay — neonatology NOW
E	Explain to patient	"My hand is keeping your baby safe."

5. Reduced Fetal Movements — KICK CHART

CAUTION — 10% of stillbirths preceded by reduced fetal movements. RESPECT MATERNAL INSTINCT. CTG first — always.

K	Kick history	When did movements decrease? Complete cessation?
I	Investigate risk factors	Post-term · hypertension · diabetes · IUGR
C	CTG — FIRST, ALWAYS	Cardiotocograph — no exceptions
K	Kick chart (if normal)	Give for home monitoring
C	Check presentation	Palpation + auscultation
H	Hand-held Doppler	If no FH on CTG
A	Amniotic fluid (AFI)	USS
R	BPP: tone + movement + breathing + fluid + CTG	5 components
T	Reassure OR Deliver	BPP ≤4 or persistent bradycardia = IMMEDIATE DELIVERY

BPP Score	CTG Finding	Action
8–10	Normal (reactive)	Reassure · discharge with kick chart
6	Non-reactive	BPP + USS — further assessment
≤4	Decelerations / bradycardia	IMMEDIATE DELIVERY

Essential Numbers — Must Know Cold

Parameter	Must Know
Severe PE threshold	≥160/110 mmHg — treat within 1 hour
Labetalol	200mg PO · 20mg IV bolus
Nifedipine	10mg PO
$MgSO_4$ loading	4g IV over 5–10 min

Parameter	Must Know
$MgSO_4$ duration	24 hours after delivery OR last seizure
$MgSO_4$ toxicity — STOP if	Loss of reflexes OR RR <12
$MgSO_4$ antidote	Calcium gluconate 1g IV
Oxytocin	10 units IM or slow IV — FIRST
Ergometrine	500 mcg IM — ✗ avoid if hypertensive
Carboprost	250 mcg IM — ✗ avoid if asthmatic
Misoprostol	800 mcg PR
Tranexamic acid	1g IV within 3 hours of delivery
Terbutaline (cord prolapse)	0.25mg SC — tocolysis
Shoulder dystocia time limit	Deliver within 5 minutes
BPP delivery threshold	≤4 or persistent bradycardia = deliver NOW
Postpartum PE window	Up to 4 weeks after delivery

One-Page Master Summary — All Emergencies

Emergency	5-Sec ID	First Action	Drug/Manoeuvre	Instant Fail
Pre-eclampsia	HTN + proteinuria >20w	ABCDE + BP control	Labetalol 200mg PO · $MgSO_4$ 4g → RARO 24h	No $MgSO_4$ · no reflex check
Eclampsia	Seizure + pre-eclampsia	Airway + $MgSO_4$ NOW	$MgSO_4$ 4g IV · Ca gluconate if toxicity	No airway protection
PPH	Postpartum + heavy bleeding	Call help + uterine massage	Oxytocin → ergometrine → carboprost → misoprostol · TXA 1g	Wrong sequence · ergometrine in HTN
Shoulder dystocia	Turtle sign + head delivered	HELPERR — NO fundal pressure	McRoberts → suprapubic → posterior arm → 5 min	FUNDAL PRESSURE
Cord prolapse	Cord visible after ROM	Hand UP — do NOT remove	Knee-chest → terbutaline → cat-1 CS	Removing hand
Reduced FMt	Mother reports decrease	CTG FIRST	USS AFI → BPP → BPP ≤4 = deliver NOW	No CTG · BPP ≤4 ignored

SBAR Handovers — All 6 Emergencies

Pre-eclampsia	S: Severe pre-eclampsia. B: BP 170/110, proteinuria 3+, headache, 36 weeks. A: Labetalol 200mg given, $MgSO_4$ 4g loading, RARO running, RR 16. R: Consultant review for delivery planning.
Eclampsia	S: Eclampsia — patient has seized. B: Known PE, 37 weeks. A: Post-ictal, airway protected, lateral tilt, $MgSO_4$ 4g given, CTG running. R: Anaesthetics + consultant URGENTLY.
PPH	S: PPH — ongoing. B: VD 20 min ago, EBL 1200 mL rising. A: 2× large-bore IV, oxytocin 10u IM, uterine massage, borderline haemodynamic. R: Consultant + anaesthetics + MHP + O-negative blood NOW.
Shoulder dystocia	S: Shoulder dystocia at delivery. B: Head delivered, turtle sign, time [X]. A: HELPERR — McRoberts + suprapubic applied, posterior arm attempted. R: Senior obstetrician + NEONATOLOGY immediately.
Cord prolapse	S: Cord prolapse — hand in situ. B: ROM 5 min ago, cord visible, fetal bradycardia. A: Hand elevating NOT removed, knee-chest, IV access, terbutaline 0.25mg SC. R: Category-1 CS NOW — anaesthetics + neonatal team to theatre.
Reduced FMt	S: Reduced fetal movements, 38 weeks. B: No movements 12h, background GDM. A: CTG non-reactive, USS reduced AFI, BPP 4. R: Consultant review — immediate delivery planning — BPP ≤4.

SAY — Must-Say Phrase Vault

Scenario	Say This
First question	“Is this mother or baby at immediate risk? MOTHER FIRST, BABY SECOND.”
RARO	“Checking reflexes, RR, urine output, GCS hourly — RARO. Loss of reflexes or RR <12 = toxicity → stop → calcium gluconate 1g IV.”
Postpartum PE	“Pre-eclampsia can occur up to 4 weeks after delivery — continuing monitoring.”
Eclampsia	“Eclampsia — airway, lateral tilt, $MgSO_4$ NOW. Calling anaesthetics.“
Uterotonics	“Sequence: oxytocin 10u IM now. BP checked → ergometrine. Asthma checked → carboprost. Misoprostol PR. TXA 1g IV.”
Shoulder — turtle sign	“Turtle sign — shoulder dystocia. DO NOT apply fundal pressure — ever.”
Shoulder — posterior arm	“Attempting posterior arm delivery — sweeping arm across chest.”
Cord — hand	“My hand is elevating the presenting part. I will NOT remove it until baby is delivered.”
BPP ≤4	“BPP ≤4 — delivering immediately. Every minute matters.”

Scenario	Say This
Maternal instinct	"You know your baby best — thank you for coming in."
Safety-net	"If movements stop completely, pain, or bleeding — come back immediately or call 999."

Examiner Checklist — All Emergencies

PE / Eclampsia ✓	PPH ✓	Shoulder · Cord ✓	RFM ✓
✓ BP ≥160/110 — 1 hour rule	✓ Buzzer activated	✓ HELPERR correct	✓ CTG performed first
✓ Labetalol/nifedipine doses	✓ Uterine massage done	✓ NO fundal pressure stated	✓ USS + BPP all 5 components
✓ $MgSO_4$ 4g IV given	✓ Oxytocin first	✓ Neonatology called	✓ BPP ≤4 = deliver NOW
✓ RARO hourly	✓ TXA 1g IV <3h	✓ Hand NOT removed (cord)	✓ Maternal instinct respected
✓ Postpartum PE (4 weeks)	✓ Ergometrine: BP checked	✓ Cat-1 CS arranged	✓ Safety-net provided
✓ Eclampsia: airway first	✓ MHP if >1500 mL		

Final Exam Mantra

MOTHER FIRST · P-PRESS · NO FUNDAL PRESSURE · NO HAND REMOVAL
CTG FIRST · $MgSO_4$ = RARO 24h · BPP ≤4 = DELIVER NOW · CALL HELP EARLY
PE up to 4 weeks postpartum · TXA 1g IV within 3h · PROTOCOL OVER THINKING
DO NOT: fundal pressure · remove hand · ergometrine in HTN · carboprost in asthma · stop $MgSO_4$ early · dismiss FMt without CTG

Mother first always, no exceptions	P-PRESS 6-emergency framework	No fundal pressure instant fail	HELPERR correct sequence	Hand UP cord never remove
MgSO4 RARO 24h reflexes + RR + urine	PE ≤4 weeks post ongoing monitoring	Oxytocin first PPH sequence	TXA 1g <3 hours mandatory in PPH	BPP ≤4 = deliver immediate action

TOP 5 EXAMINER Q&A · O&G EMERGENCIES

Q1. Eclamptic seizure: drug and dose?	Magnesium sulfate 4 g IV over 5–15 minutes then infusion: plus left lateral position, airway protection and urgent obstetric/anaesthetic help.
Q2. The 4 Ts of postpartum haemorrhage?	Tone, trauma, tissue, thrombin: massage the uterus, give uterotonics, and activate the major haemorrhage protocol early.

TOP 5 EXAMINER Q&A · O&G EMERGENCIES	
Q3. Shoulder dystocia: first manoeuvres?	Call for help, McRoberts position, suprapubic pressure: state the manoeuvres aloud and note the time.
Q4. Cord prolapse: immediate actions?	Relieve pressure off the cord (elevate presenting part, knee-chest position), do not handle the cord, category 1 caesarean.
Q5. Severe pre-eclampsia: blood pressure treatment?	IV labetalol (or alternatives) targeting below 135/85, with magnesium prophylaxis considered and senior obstetric care.
CURVEBALL	A collapsed postnatal woman with heavy lochia and a boggy uterus. Treat tone first while resuscitating: bimanual compression, uterotonics, major haemorrhage call: simultaneously, not sequentially.

CHAPTER 44 · O&G III: POSTPARTUM COMPLICATIONS

Breastfeeding · Perinatal Mental Health

POST-BIRTH · RETAINED · CLOT · HEAD · SEPSIS · 3 Bs · SAD MOM · PSYCHOSIS

HIGH · GREEN · YELLOW PATH · CAUTION — MODERATE INSTANT FAIL RISK

Abbreviations used in this chapter: **CBT** Cognitive Behavioural Therapy · **COCP** Combined Oral Contraceptive Pill · **CTPA** CT Pulmonary Angiogram · **DVT** Deep Vein Thrombosis · **EPDS** Edinburgh Postnatal Depression Scale · **ERPC** Evacuation of Retained Products of Conception · **IUD** Intrauterine Device · **IUS** Intrauterine System · **LMWH** Low Molecular Weight Heparin · **MDT** Multidisciplinary Team · **PE** Pulmonary Embolism · **POP** Progestogen-Only Pill · **PPH** Postpartum Haemorrhage · **RUQ** Right Upper Quadrant · **TXA** Tranexamic Acid · **USS** Ultrasound Scan · **VTE** Venous Thromboembolism

THINK — Core Rule: BIG FOUR first — every postpartum patient: Bleeding · Sepsis · VTE · Pre-eclampsia.
First Question: "What is the timing — immediate (<24h), early (24h–7d), or late (>7d)?"

SAY — Golden Minute: "I'll check physical red flags first — bleeding, infection, clots, blood pressure — then emotional wellbeing, then feeding and bonding."

POST-BIRTH — 9-Complication Recall

P	Psychosis	EMERGENCY — MBU + safeguarding NOW
O	Ongoing bleeding (secondary PPH)	USS → ERPC + TXA 1g
S	Sepsis	Sepsis Six → IV antibiotics within 1h
T	Thrombosis (VTE)	LMWH immediately — no D-dimer
B	Breast problems	Mastitis → flucloxacillin 500mg QDS → continue feeding
I	Increased BP	Postpartum pre-eclampsia → HEAD mnemonic
R	Retention (urinary)	Bladder scan → catheterise
T	Tears/wound infection	Inspect → swab → antibiotics
H	Home support & mental health	EPDS ≥13 → treat → perinatal team

Instant Fail Triggers

Missed sepsis (fever called normal) · Missed VTE (chest pain dismissed) · D-dimer used postpartum
Missed postpartum pre-eclampsia · Psychosis missed or not escalated · No safeguarding referral
Low mood dismissed as baby blues · Discharged without safety-net or follow-up

1. Secondary PPH · VTE

Secondary PPH: Bleeding >24h postpartum = secondary PPH until proven otherwise. Act on clinical suspicion.

	RETAINED (Causes)	**Action**
R	Retained products	USS → ERPC if confirmed
E	Endometritis	Antibiotics
T	Trauma	Inspect genital tract
A	Atony	Uterine massage
I	Infection	Broad-spectrum IV antibiotics
N	No clotting (coagulopathy)	Coag screen
E	Evacuation (ERPC)	If retained products confirmed
D	Delayed = danger	Act early

VTE: Postpartum chest pain / SOB / calf pain = VTE until proven otherwise.
CLOT: Calf swelling · Leg pain · Out of breath · Tachycardia
Do NOT use D-dimer postpartum — always elevated. Clinical suspicion = start LMWH immediately.
PE: Enoxaparin 1mg/kg SC BD → CTPA (safe — continue breastfeeding after scan)
DVT: Compression USS → LMWH if confirmed

2. Postnatal Sepsis · Postpartum Pre-eclampsia

Sepsis: Postpartum fever = sepsis until proven otherwise — do NOT dismiss as normal.

	SEPSIS Sources	**Sepsis Six — Within 1 Hour**
S	Section wound	1. Oxygen
E	Endometritis	2. Blood cultures before antibiotics
P	Perineal wound	3. Broad-spectrum IV antibiotics
S	Sepsis from UTI	4. IV fluids if unstable
I	Infected breast	5. Lactate
S	Systemic (retained products)	6. Urine output monitoring

HEAD — Postpartum Pre-eclampsia (up to 4 WEEKS post-delivery):
H — Headache (severe) · E — Elevated BP (≥160/110) · A — Abdominal pain (RUQ) · D — Disturbed vision
Actions: BP → labetalol 200mg PO / 20mg IV or nifedipine 10mg PO → $MgSO_4$ 4g if severe → RARO → obstetric review
SAY — Must-Say: "Do NOT dismiss headache as tension in a postnatal patient — check BP first."

3. Retention · Wound · Mastitis · Contraception

Condition	Management
Urinary retention	Ask about voiding · bladder scan · catheterise if confirmed
Perineal wound	Inspect · swab · antibiotics · analgesia. Red flag: incontinence of stool/wind → sphincter injury → perineal clinic
Mastitis	Flucloxacillin 500mg QDS 10–14 days · CONTINUE feeding — stopping worsens mastitis · USS at 48h if not improving
Breast abscess	USS confirms → aspiration or drainage · continue antibiotics. Not resolving → breast clinic (exclude cancer)

Contraception	Breastfeeding	Non-breastfeeding
POP / Implant / IUS	Safe — start immediately	Safe — start immediately
COCP	✗ Avoid until 6 weeks	Can start at 21 days
Condoms / Copper IUD	Safe any time	Safe any time

THINK — 4. Perinatal Mental Health — 3 Bs · SAD MOM · PSYCHOSIS

3 Bs	Condition	Timing	Action
Blues	Baby Blues	Days 3–10	Mild, weepy — REASSURE ONLY — no treatment
Blow	Postnatal Depression (PND)	Weeks 2–52	EPDS ≥13 → sertraline 50mg OD (safe in breastfeeding) · CBT · perinatal team
Bizarre	Postpartum Psychosis	Days 3–14	EMERGENCY — MBU + safeguarding NOW

SAD MOM — PND Red Flags:
S — Sleep disturbance · A — Anhedonia · D — Depressed mood · M — Mum-baby bonding · O — Overwhelmed · M — Morbid thoughts (harm to self or baby)
PND Screen: EPDS ≥13 = probable PND → refer to perinatal mental health team → sertraline 50mg OD + CBT
Safety: "Any thoughts of harming yourself or your baby?" — must ask every time

PSYCHOSIS — PSYCHIATRIC EMERGENCY (Days 3–14):

Paranoia · Sleep loss (days) · Confusion/disorganised speech · Command hallucinations · Rapid onset · Risk to self AND baby

Actions: Call psychiatric emergency team · Do NOT leave alone with baby · Emergency MBU admission · Safeguarding referral NOW

SAY — Must-Say: "This is a psychiatric emergency — safety of mother and baby is my priority. Calling psychiatric team now."

Safeguarding · MDT · Admit vs Outpatient

Safeguarding — always speak to mother ALONE:

"How are things at home? Do you feel safe?" · Observe mother-infant interaction · Document factually · Escalate if concerns

Red flags: Inconsistent history · unexplained injuries · mother frightened · controlling partner · poor bonding

Admit	Outpatient / Community
Sepsis	Mild mastitis + antibiotics
Secondary PPH (unstable)	Baby blues
Pre-eclampsia / eclampsia	Mild PND (safety confirmed)
Confirmed VTE	Breastfeeding / contraception advice
Postpartum psychosis	
Safeguarding concerns	

Examiner Checklist

BIG FOUR: ✓ Bleeding assessed · ✓ Sepsis Six if fever · ✓ VTE — no D-dimer, LMWH started · ✓ BP + urine dip

Physical: ✓ Voiding asked · ✓ Perineum inspected · ✓ Mastitis: flucloxacillin 500mg QDS stated, feeding continued · ✓ Contraception: COCP avoided <6 weeks breastfeeding

Mental health: ✓ 3 Bs distinguished · ✓ EPDS ≥13 = treat · ✓ Sertraline 50mg safe in breastfeeding stated · ✓ Psychosis = MBU + safeguarding

Communication: ✓ Spoke ALONE · ✓ Safety question asked · ✓ Safety-net given · ✓ Follow-up arranged

Final Exam Mantra

BIG FOUR first: Bleeding · Sepsis · VTE (no D-dimer, LMWH) · Pre-eclampsia (HEAD, up to 4 weeks)

Mastitis: flucloxacillin 500mg QDS · continue feeding · USS at 48h

3 Bs: Blues=reassure / Blow=EPDS ≥13 + sertraline 50mg / Bizarre=MBU + safeguarding NOW

Speak ALONE · Ask "Do you feel safe?" · CTPA safe in breastfeeding · Safety-net always

Gold Closing:
"I've ruled out THE BIG FOUR. We've assessed physical health, mental health, feeding, and bonding. Treatment and referrals are in place. If you develop fever, chest pain, heavy bleeding, severe headache, or thoughts of harming yourself or your baby — call immediately."

BIG FOUR first bleed·sepsis·VTE·BP	No D-dimer postpartum always elevated	LMWH 1mg/kg BD VTE treatment	Fluclox 500mg QDS 10-14 days mastitis	Continue feeding mastitis rule
EPDS ≥13 = treat PND threshold	Sertraline 50mg safe breastfeeding safe	3 Bs framework blues/blow/bizarre	Psychosis = MBU NOW not alone + safeguard	HEAD up to 4 weeks postpartum PE

TOP 5 EXAMINER Q&A · POSTPARTUM COMPLICATIONS	
Q1. Mastitis in a breastfeeding mother: key advice?	Continue feeding or expressing from the affected breast; antibiotics if systemically unwell or not settling: abscess needs ultrasound.
Q2. Baby blues vs postnatal depression?	Blues peak around day 3–5 and resolve by two weeks; persistent low mood, anhedonia or functional decline beyond that is depression: screen and treat.
Q3. Which postnatal presentation is a psychiatric emergency?	Postpartum psychosis: confusion, mood swings, delusions about the baby: same-day specialist assessment, usually admission.
Q4. Fever at day 5 postpartum: what must you cover?	Endometritis, wound and breast infection, UTI and VTE: examine all sites and treat sepsis promptly.
Q5. What must every perinatal mental health assessment include?	Thoughts of self-harm and thoughts of harming the baby, asked directly and without judgement.
CURVEBALL	She admits intrusive thoughts of dropping the baby and is horrified by them. Distinguish intrusive thoughts (common, ego-dystonic) from intent: assess risk carefully: horror at the thought is usually reassuring.

CHAPTER 45 · O&G IV: SEXUAL ASSAULT, FGM, TERMINATION & SAFEGUARDING

SAFE-CARE · FORCE · C.E.I.O. · PAINS · BRAIN · FRASER · GROUNDS A–E

CORE · GREEN PATH · CAUTION — CRITICAL INSTANT FAIL RISK

Abbreviations used in this chapter: FGM Female Genital Mutilation · **FSRH** Faculty of Sexual & Reproductive Healthcare · **IUD** Intrauterine Device · **SARC** Sexual Assault Referral Centre

THINK — First Question — Every Station: "Is this a safeguarding issue? Do I have a mandatory duty to report?"
Examiner Mindset: "If you don't escalate a safeguarding concern, I fail you."

SAY — Golden Minute: "Using SAFE-CARE: Safeguarding first — is anyone at risk? Assess scenario — assault, FGM, TOP, or abuse? Follow the law — mandatory duty? Explain, Communicate, Act immediately — refer, treat, escalate. Record verbatim. Escalate to safeguarding lead, social services, or police."

SAFE-CARE — Master Framework (Every O&G Scenario)

S	Safeguarding first	Is anyone at risk? Child? Vulnerable adult?
A	Assess scenario	Assault? FGM? TOP? Abuse?
F	Follow the law	Mandatory reporting? Abortion Act grounds?
E	Explain to patient	Transparency builds trust and marks
C	Communicate empathetically	Non-judgmental, patient-centred
A	Act immediately	Refer, escalate, treat — no delays
R	Record meticulously	Verbatim, body map, chain of evidence
E	Escalate	Safeguarding lead, social services, police

Instant Fail Triggers

No SARC referral · No EC offered (especially Cu-IUD) · Clothes in plastic bag (destroys DNA)
FGM under-18 not reported to police · Safeguarding concern not escalated · Child sent home at risk
Promising secrecy to child · Conscientious objection without referral · No Fraser competence under-16
No pregnancy test (baseline + 3 weeks) · HIV PEP window missed · Daughters under-18 not asked in FGM

Station Recognition · Essential Numbers

If you see...	Think...
Assault disclosure <72h	FORCE + SARC + EC + PEP + paper bag

If you see...	Think...
Antenatal + FGM-practising country	C.E.I.O. + deinfibulate + check daughters
Termination request	BRAIN + Abortion Act + check coercion
Child disclosure or injury	Verbatim + body map + escalate immediately
Under-16 requesting contraception/TOP	Fraser competence + safeguard if risk
Colleague refuses TOP patient	Conscientious objection — must refer NOW

Parameter	Threshold / Action
Levonelle	Within 72 hours
EllaOne	Within 120 hours — safe in breastfeeding (2025 FSRH — no interruption needed)
Cu-IUD	MOST EFFECTIVE — within 5 days (or 5d post-ovulation)
HIV PEP	Start within 72h — ideally under 24h
FGM mandatory report	Under-18 — police by next working day
TOP time limit	24 weeks for most grounds (Ground C)
TOP Ground E	Severe fetal abnormality — NO time limit
Pregnancy test	Baseline now + repeat at 3 weeks post-assault

1. Sexual Assault — FORCE Framework

	FORCE	Action	Must-Say
F	Forensic evidence	PAPER BAG for clothes — NEVER plastic. Assess immediate injuries FIRST. Do NOT examine before SARC.	"Clothes in paper bag — never plastic."
O	Offer EC + prophylaxis	Cu-IUD = MOST EFFECTIVE <5d. EllaOne <120h (safe breastfeeding). Levonelle <72h. HIV PEP <72h. Hep B + STI antibiotics.	"Cu-IUD is the most effective option."
R	Reporting	Police: discuss, not mandatory for adults. Under-18 = mandatory safeguarding referral. Self-referral to SARC available.	"You can self-refer if not ready for police."
C	Consent	Meticulous written consent for every step. Patient controls every part.	"Your consent at every step."

	FORCE	Action	Must-Say
E	Emotional support	SARC follow-up, counselling, safe discharge, capacity check.	"SARC has specially trained staff."

Common Traps:
Plastic bag → destroys DNA · Multiple retellings → contaminates evidence · Missing Cu-IUD as best EC · Old EllaOne breastfeeding advice (2025: no interruption needed)

2. FGM — C.E.I.O. + PAINS

	Type	Name	Description
C	Type I	Clitoridectomy	Partial or total removal of clitoris
E	Type II	Excision	Removal of clitoris + labia minora
I	Type III	Infibulation	Narrowing of vaginal opening + sealing labia → deinfibulation needed
O	Type IV	Other	Pricking, burning, or other harmful procedures

PAINS — Complications:
P — Pain (acute + chronic) · A — Anxiety/psychological trauma · I — Infections (UTI, STI) · N — Narrowing (obstructed labour, tears) · S — Sexual dysfunction

Legal Duties:
Performing / assisting FGM = ILLEGAL · Taking child abroad for FGM = ILLEGAL (FGM Act 2003)
Under-18 disclosure → MANDATORY report to police by NEXT WORKING DAY
Re-infibulation after delivery = ILLEGAL — no clinical justification
SAY — Must-Say: "Do you have any daughters under 18, either here in the UK or abroad?"
SAY — Sensitive ask: "Sometimes women from communities where FGM is practised have had some cutting — is that something that happened to you?"

3. Termination of Pregnancy (TOP) — BRAIN + Grounds A–E

	BRAIN	Script
B	Benefits	"A termination would mean you are no longer pregnant."
R	Risks	"Small risk of infection, bleeding, or failure."
A	Alternatives	"Continue the pregnancy and keep the baby, or adoption."
I	Intuition	"How are you feeling about this?"
N	Next steps	"You don't have to decide now. Let's talk through what happens next."

Ground	Indication	Time Limit
A	Risk to life of pregnant person	Any gestation

Ground	Indication	Time Limit
B	Prevent grave permanent injury	Any gestation
C	Risk to physical/mental health (MOST COMMON)	<24 weeks
D	Risk to health of existing children	<24 weeks
E	Substantial risk of serious fetal abnormality	NO TIME LIMIT

Two doctors must sign. Medical (early pregnancy) and surgical options both available. Coercion check: "I want to check this decision is yours — are you feeling pressured by anyone?"

Conscientious Objection:
"Due to my personal beliefs I cannot arrange this. However, I will immediately refer you to a colleague who will see you right away. I will not leave you without support."
✗ Cannot refuse without arranging alternative · ✗ Cannot judge or lecture · ✓ Must provide emergency care regardless

4. Fraser Competence (Under-16) · Vulnerable Adults

Fraser Competence — All 6 criteria must be YES to proceed without parental consent:
1. Understands advice + implications · 2. Mature enough to decide independently · 3. In their best interests
4. Free from coercion · 5. Understands risks of NOT receiving care · 6. Will engage with services
If any = NO → involve safeguarding. Document assessment VERBATIM.

Vulnerable Adults: Assess capacity (understand · retain · weigh · communicate). If lacking capacity + at risk → safeguarding referral MANDATORY. Decisions follow best-interest principles.
Screen for: Coercion · domestic abuse · honour-based violence · exploitation

5. Safeguarding · Verbatim Documentation

Rule: Listen → Document verbatim → Body map → NEVER promise secrecy → Escalate immediately.
SAY — To child: "Thank you for telling me. I need to tell someone whose job is to keep children safe — I won't tell everyone, but I must tell the people who can help."
Immediate danger → CALL 999. Do NOT send child home at risk.

Abuse Category	Features
Physical	Bruises, fractures, burns — inconsistent with history
Sexual	Genital injury, inappropriate behaviour, STIs, disclosure
Neglect	Hunger, poor hygiene, untreated medical needs, poor growth

Escalation Pathway:

1. Discuss with safeguarding lead — in hours · 2. Immediate risk → social services / police NOW
3. Child in immediate danger → do NOT leave → call 999 · 4. Document: who, when, what agreed

SBAR: "Escalating urgently to safeguarding lead. Situation: child disclosure of abuse. Assessment: immediate risk. Recommendation: social services + police."

Examiner Checklist

Sexual Assault + FGM ✓	TOP + Safeguarding + Under-16 ✓
✓ Immediate injuries assessed first	✓ BRAIN used — non-judgmental
✓ Paper bag — NOT plastic	✓ Abortion Act grounds stated (C most common, E no limit)
✓ SARC referral + self-referral option	✓ Coercion checked
✓ Cu-IUD offered as most effective EC	✓ Conscientious objection: referral arranged
✓ EllaOne: safe breastfeeding (2025)	✓ Fraser competence: all 6 criteria
✓ HIV PEP <72h discussed	✓ Fraser assessment documented verbatim
✓ Baseline + 3-week pregnancy test	✓ Listened without interrupting
✓ C.E.I.O. classification used	✓ Verbatim documentation + body map
✓ Type III → deinfibulation explained	✓ Did NOT promise confidentiality to child
✓ Daughters under-18 asked	✓ Child NOT sent home at risk
✓ Under-18 FGM → police by next working day	✓ 999 if immediate danger
✓ Re-infibulation stated as illegal	✓ Escalated via SBAR

Final Exam Mantra

SAFE-CARE first · FORCE for assault · PAPER BAG not plastic · Cu-IUD = best EC · EllaOne safe breastfeeding (2025)

C.E.I.O. for FGM · PAINS complications · Daughters under-18 · Under-18 FGM = police by next working day

BRAIN for TOP · Ground C <24w · Ground E no limit · Conscientious objection = refer immediately

Fraser: all 6 criteria · Verbatim + body map · Never promise secrecy · 999 if immediate danger

Gold Closing:

"Using SAFE-CARE: safeguarding checked first, scenario assessed, legal duties followed, patient informed, empathetic communication throughout, acted immediately with referrals and treatment, recorded verbatim, and escalated to the appropriate team. Safety-netting provided."

SAFE-CARE master framework	Paper bag never plastic	Cu-IUD = best EC within 5 days	EllaOne safe BF 2025 FSRH	HIV PEP <72h ideally <24h
FGM under-18 police next day	Re-infibulation illegal always	Ground C <24w most common TOP	Ground E no time limit	Fraser: all 6 document verbatim

TOP 5 EXAMINER Q&A · SEXUAL ASSAULT, FGM, TERMINATION & SAFEGUARDING	
Q1. First priorities for a person disclosing sexual assault?	Safety, belief and choice: address injuries, offer SARC referral, preserve forensic evidence, and follow their decisions.
Q2. What time-critical interventions do you offer?	Emergency contraception, HIV post-exposure prophylaxis (within 72 hours), hepatitis B vaccination and STI screening.
Q3. Your legal duty when you identify FGM in an under-18?	Mandatory reporting to the police, alongside safeguarding referral: explain the duty sensitively.
Q4. Grounds for termination under the Abortion Act?	Most are Ground C before 24 weeks; two doctors' signatures; conscientious objection never permits obstructing referral.
Q5. How do you safeguard without breaking trust?	Be honest about the limits of confidentiality from the start: explain what you must share, with whom and why.
CURVEBALL	An adult patient discloses assault but refuses police involvement. Her choice governs: document factually, offer SARC self-referral (which preserves evidence without police), and leave the door open.

CHAPTER 46 · SUBFERTILITY & INITIAL WORKUP

SPAT · Both Partners · Referral Criteria · Inclusive Care
Semen Analysis · Progesterone · AMH · Tubal Patency · Lifestyle
VERY HIGH · GREEN PATH · CAUTION — HIGH INSTANT FAIL RISK

Abbreviations used in this chapter: **AMH** Anti-Mullerian Hormone · **FSH** Follicle-Stimulating Hormone · **HSG** Hysterosalpingogram · **IVF** In Vitro Fertilisation · **LMP** Last Menstrual Period · **MMR** Measles, Mumps & Rubella · **NTD** Neural Tube Defect · **PID** Pelvic Inflammatory Disease

THINK — Core Rule: Investigate BOTH partners simultaneously. SPAT in parallel. Tubal patency ONLY after normal semen AND negative chlamydia. >35 = refer at 6 months — never wait 12.
First Question: "Is this unexplained, anovulatory, male factor, or tubal?"
Examiner Mindset: "If you don't investigate both partners simultaneously, I fail you."

SAY — Golden Minute: "Subfertility is defined as not conceiving after one year of regular unprotected intercourse (every 2–3 days). We investigate both partners simultaneously — it takes two to conceive. SPAT: Semen analysis, Progesterone, AMH in parallel from day one — tubal patency only after semen normal and chlamydia negative."

SPAT — Core Investigation Framework

S	Semen analysis (male)	3 days abstinence · repeat once after 3 months if abnormal	Start from day 1 — run in parallel
P	Progesterone (female)	7 days before expected period (mid-luteal)	Confirms ovulation
A	AMH (female)	Any time in cycle · ovarian reserve	Guides treatment timing
T	Tubal patency (female)	HSG or HyCoSy	ONLY after: semen normal + chlamydia negative

Instant Fail Triggers

Female-only investigation (male factor in 30% of cases) · Waiting 12 months if female >35
Tubal test without chlamydia screen first · Tubal test before semen result
Advising IVF without completing workup · Dismissing single/same-sex patients
Forgetting rubella check · Missing red flags (galactorrhoea, hot flushes, ED)

Essential Numbers — Must Know

Parameter	**Threshold / Action**
Referral — age <35	Trying 12 months → refer
Referral — age >35	Trying 6 months → refer NOW — do NOT wait

Parameter	Threshold / Action
Immediate referral	Known cause (azoospermia, amenorrhoea, ectopic, PID, high FSH, chemo) or same-sex/single
Progesterone timing	7 days before next expected period
Semen analysis	3 days abstinence · repeat once after 3 months if abnormal
BMI target	19–25 · IVF requires BMI <30
Folic acid — standard	400 mcg daily
Folic acid — high dose	5 mg daily: diabetes · epilepsy · BMI >30 · family history NTD
Rubella	Check IgG · vaccinate if non-immune · avoid pregnancy 1 month after MMR
Intercourse frequency	Every 2–3 days — NOT daily targeting ovulation

1. History — Both Partners (Never Female-Only)

Female Partner	Key Questions
Menstrual	Cycle length (21–35 days normal)? Regular? LMP?
Obstetric	Previous pregnancies? Miscarriages? Ectopics?
Gynaecological	PID? STIs? Endometriosis? Fibroids?
Surgical	Pelvic surgery? Appendicectomy? Ovarian cyst?
Medications	ACE inhibitors · statins · NSAIDs · retinoids → stop if trying to conceive
Contraception	Prior IUDs/implants? When stopped?

Male Partner	Key Questions
Reproductive	Previous children (current or other partners)?
Sexual function	Erectile dysfunction? Ejaculatory problems?
Medical/surgical	Undescended testes? Mumps post-puberty? Hernia repair?
Medications	Anabolic steroids? Sulfasalazine?
Occupational	Heat exposure? Toxins?

Red Flags — Do Not Miss:
Galactorrhoea → check prolactin · Hot flushes + amenorrhoea → FSH (ovarian insufficiency → refer immediately)
Erectile dysfunction → check hormones · Testicular atrophy/gynaecomastia → LH/FSH/testosterone

2. SPAT Investigations in Detail

Test	Detail
Semen analysis	3 days abstinence. Assesses count, motility, morphology. Repeat once after 3 months if abnormal. Lifestyle review + urology if still abnormal.
Progesterone	7 days before next expected period (mid-luteal). Confirms ovulation. Irregular cycles → serial testing.
AMH	Any time in cycle. Low AMH = reduced ovarian reserve → earlier referral. Guides treatment decisions.
Tubal patency	HSG or HyCoSy. MUST have ALL THREE first: ovulation confirmed + semen normal + chlamydia negative. If abnormal → refer for laparoscopy / IVF.
Rubella IgG	Vaccinate if non-immune (MMR). Avoid pregnancy 1 month after vaccination.
Chlamydia screen	BEFORE tubal tests. Chlamydia may be asymptomatic. Tubal test can flare PID if active infection.
TSH + prolactin	If irregular cycles or galactorrhoea.
FSH	If irregular cycles or suspected ovarian insufficiency. High FSH → refer immediately.

TIP — 3. Lifestyle Advice · Referral Criteria

Factor	Advice
Smoking	Stop — single most important factor. Refer to NHS Stop Smoking Services.
BMI	Target 19–25. BMI >30 → weight management. IVF requires <30. BMI <19 → dietitian.
Folic acid	400 mcg daily standard. 5 mg if: diabetes · epilepsy · BMI >30 · family history NTD.
Intercourse	Every 2–3 days throughout cycle — regular is better than targeting fertile window.
Medications	Stop ACE inhibitors · statins · NSAIDs · retinoids if trying to conceive.
Lubricants	Some reduce sperm movement — use fertility-friendly brand if needed.
Alcohol	<14 units/week both partners. No binge drinking.

Referral Rules:

<35 years: routine referral after 12 months · >35 years: refer at 6 months — DO NOT WAIT

Immediate referral: azoospermia · amenorrhoea · previous ectopic/PID · chemo/RT · high FSH · same-sex/single patients

4. Inclusive Care

Patient	Pathway
Same-sex female couple	Same SPAT for carrying partner. Refer for donor insemination. Both partners involved throughout.
Same-sex male couple	Refer for surrogacy + egg donation. Semen analysis for intended father(s).
Single woman	Same initial workup as a couple. Entitled to IUI or IVF with donor sperm.

Common Scenarios:
8 months trying (<35): "Still within normal. No referral yet. Starting SPAT + lifestyle today."
37-year-old, 11 months: "Because of your age, referring to fertility clinic now and starting tests while you wait."
Abnormal semen: "Common finding. Repeating in 3 months. Reviewing lifestyle and considering urology."

Examiner Checklist

History + Investigations ✓	Lifestyle + Referral ✓
✓ Both partners asked	✓ Smoking cessation advised
✓ Menstrual + obstetric history	✓ BMI addressed (target 19–25, IVF <30)
✓ Male reproductive + sexual function	✓ Folic acid: standard or 5mg high-dose stated
✓ Duration trying + frequency established	✓ Medications reviewed
✓ SPAT explained in parallel	✓ Intercourse every 2–3 days
✓ Progesterone timing correct (7d before period)	✓ Referral criteria: 12 vs 6 months stated
✓ Tubal pre-requisites stated	✓ >35 referred at 6 months
✓ Chlamydia before tubal test	✓ Immediate referral triggers identified
✓ Rubella IgG checked	✓ Inclusive care: same-sex/single managed
✓ Red flags addressed	✓ Safety-net + follow-up 3–6 months

Final Exam Mantra

BOTH partners · SPAT in parallel · T only after normal S + negative chlamydia · >35 = 6 months not 12
Folic acid 400mcg (or 5mg high-risk) · BMI 19–25 · Smoking = single most important factor
Rubella IgG · Inclusive care · Immediate referral for known causes · Safety-net 3–6 months

Gold Closing:
"I've taken a comprehensive history from both of you. SPAT investigations are arranged in parallel. Tubal patency will follow once semen and chlamydia results are available. Lifestyle advice given: smoking, BMI, folic acid, medication review, intercourse every 2–3 days. Referral criteria met/discussed. Follow-up in 3–6 months."

Both partners always simultaneously	SPAT in parallel S+P+A from day 1	T only after normal S + neg chlamydia	>35 = 6 months never wait 12	Progesterone 7 days before period
Folic acid 400mcg 5mg if high-risk	Smoking = #1 refer to stop smoking	BMI 19–25 IVF requires <30	Rubella IgG vaccinate if needed	Immediate refer known cause always

TOP 5 EXAMINER Q&A · SUBFERTILITY & INITIAL WORKUP	
Q1. When does subfertility investigation begin?	After 12 months of regular unprotected intercourse: earlier if she is 36 or over or there are known risk factors.
Q2. What does the initial couple workup include?	Both partners from the start: semen analysis, mid-luteal progesterone, cycle history, chlamydia screening and lifestyle review.
Q3. How do you confirm ovulation?	Mid-luteal (day 21 in a 28-day cycle) serum progesterone, timed to her actual cycle length.
Q4. Abnormal semen analysis: next step?	Repeat in three months before referral: counsel sensitively; avoid blame framing.
Q5. Which lifestyle factors genuinely matter?	Smoking, alcohol, BMI extremes and timing of intercourse: optimise both partners while investigating.
CURVEBALL	The couple has been trying for 8 months and is distressed. Validate without premature investigation: explain normal timelines, optimise lifestyle, and agree a clear review point: managing expectation is the skill.

CHAPTER 47 · PAEDS I: FEBRILE CHILD, SEPSIS & MENINGOCOCCAL DISEASE

SICK RASH · RASH · STIFF · CRASH+BURN · WET · Traffic Light · ABCDE

CORE · RED PATH · CAUTION — HIGH INSTANT FAIL RISK

Abbreviations used in this chapter: **AVPU** Alert, Voice, Pain, Unresponsive · **BNF** British National Formulary · **CRT** Capillary Refill Time · **LP** Lumbar Puncture

THINK — Core Rule: Examiners want safety thinking, NOT detail. Recognise sick child early · ABCDE · oxygen + fluids + antibiotics fast · escalate · safety-net.

4 Non-Negotiables: 1. ABCDE 2. Check CRT 3. Glass test for rash 4. Oxygen + 10 ml/kg fluids + antibiotics within 1 hour

Anchor: "Oxygen + position of comfort first — even if unsure of exact scenario."

SAY — Golden Minute: "Well or sick? Green, amber, or red? Non-blanching rash = IM benzylpenicillin NOW. 10 ml/kg — not 5. Antibiotics within 1 hour. Stop → Treat → Escalate → Reassess."

SICK RASH — All Red Flags (Master Mnemonic)

S	Shock (CRT ≥3 sec, tachycardia)	Fluid bolus 10 ml/kg — NOT 5	Reassess after every bolus
I	Irritable / inconsolable	Escalate immediately	AVPU <A = PICU
C	Cyanosed / mottled	Oxygen + escalate	
K	Keeps vomiting / poor feeding	Consider sepsis	
R	Rash non-blanching	IM benzylpenicillin NOW	Glass test — must verbalise
A	Altered consciousness (AVPU <A)	Escalate to PICU	
S	Stridor / severe resp distress	Position of comfort · senior NOW	Epiglottitis: DO NOT examine throat
H	High RR (>60) or hypoxia	Oxygen · assess immediately	

Automatic Red Flags — No Thinking Delay:
Fever <3 months → URGENT referral · Silent chest + exhaustion → PICU NOW · Tripod + drooling + toxic → EPIGLOTTITIS — call anaesthetics, DO NOT examine throat

NICE Traffic Light · ABCDE Dual-Track

Colour	Key Features	Action
GREEN	Happy · hydrated · interactive · normal colour	Home with two-layer safety-netting

Colour	Key Features	Action
AMBER	Tired · tachycardic · reduced feeding · CRT ≥3 sec	Senior review · investigations · observe
RED	Lethargic · mottled/cyanosed · non-blanching rash · grunting · seizure · <3 months fever	URGENT — ABCDE + fluids + antibiotics

Viral vs Bacterial Quick Check:
Viral: Gradual onset · normal colour · playful · Bacterial: Sudden · pale/mottled · lethargic · CRT ≥3 sec · possible non-blanching rash

Instant Fail Triggers

Missing non-blanching rash · Delay IM benzylpenicillin for IV access · Give 5 ml/kg bolus (must be 10)
Examine throat in epiglottitis · Send home a red traffic light child · No senior involvement
Antipyretics to prevent seizures (comfort only) · No urine dip (fever without source) · Ignore parental concern

1. Meningococcal Disease · Meningitis — RASH · STIFF

RASH: Rapid onset · Appears ill (toxic) · Spots non-blanching · Haemorrhagic/purpuric
STIFF: Stiff neck · Trouble with light (photophobia) · Irritable · Fontanelle bulging · Fever
SAY — Glass test: "Rash does not blanch — treating as meningococcal disease until proven otherwise."

IM Benzylpenicillin Doses — Must Know:
<1 year: 300mg · 1–9 years: 600mg · ≥10 years/adults: 1.2g · Give IM immediately if IV access difficult — DO NOT WAIT.

Step	Action	Detail
1	ABCDE	Verbalise every finding
2	Oxygen	High-flow if hypoxic
3	IM benzylpenicillin	If IV access difficult — give NOW, do NOT wait
4	IV antibiotics within 1 hour	<3 months: cefotaxime + amoxicillin · ≥3 months: ceftriaxone
5	Fluid bolus 10 ml/kg	If shocked — reassess CRT + HR after every bolus
6	Urgent transfer	SBAR handover before transfer

Do NOT LP if: Reduced consciousness · focal neurology · papilloedema · seizure <30 min · cardiovascular instability

2. Kawasaki · UTI · Febrile Seizure · WET Dehydration

CRASH + BURN — Kawasaki:
C — Conjunctivitis (bilateral, non-exudative) · R — Rash (polymorphous) · A — Adenopathy (cervical) · S — Strawberry tongue · H — Hands/feet erythema + oedema
BURN — Fever >5 days: diagnostic trigger. Risk: coronary artery aneurysms. Can mimic sepsis. Urgent paediatric referral.

Feature	Simple Febrile Seizure	Complex Febrile Seizure
Duration	<15 minutes	>15 minutes
Type	Generalised	Focal
Recurrence	Once in 24h	>1 in 24h
Action	Discharge + safety-net	Admit + investigate

Antipyretics: DO NOT prevent febrile seizures — for COMFORT ONLY. Never advise parents otherwise.

WET — Dehydration Assessment:
W — Wet nappies <4 in 24h · E — Eyes sunken · T — Tears absent + fontanelle sunken
Treat: Oral rehydration (small frequent sips) · IV fluids if severe · NG if <50% normal intake

Fever Without Source — Always Do:
Urine dip (UTI = most common cause <3 years) · Consider Kawasaki if fever >5 days · Check immunisation status

3. Respiratory Emergencies — Quick Reference

Scenario	Flash Trigger	Critical Action	Urgency
Stridor + barking cough + well	CROUP	Oral dexamethasone · neb adrenaline if severe · admit if stridor at rest	AMBER
Stridor + drooling + tripod + toxic	EPIGLOTTITIS	DO NOT examine throat · position of comfort · call anaesthetics NOW	RED
Wheeze + asthma + silent chest	ASTHMA	Salbutamol spacer · reassess · escalate if silent chest	AMBER/RED
Infant <1yr + coryza + wheeze	BRONCHIOLITIS	Oxygen if SpO_2 <92% · NO bronchodilators · supportive	AMBER
Sudden choking + coughing	FOREIGN BODY	Age-appropriate manoeuvre · senior	RED
Rapid rash + hypotension + stridor	ANAPHYLAXIS	IM adrenaline 1:1000 · high-flow O_2 · call crash team	RED

SAY — Parent Communication · SBAR · Admit vs Discharge

Two-Layer Safety-Netting:

Primary: "If breathing worsens or feeding drops, return immediately."

Emergency: "Rash that doesn't fade · stops drinking · fewer wet nappies · drowsy · seizure → call 999 immediately."

Instinct: "Trust your instinct — if worried, come back."

Empathy: "You did the right thing bringing them in. I can see this is frightening — we're acting quickly."

Antipyretics: "For comfort only — will not prevent seizures. Hydration is more important than the temperature number."

SBAR — 30-Second Script:

S: "[Age] child with fever and features of sepsis."

B: "Fever [X]h · immunisations [status] · wet nappies [number] · traffic light: [colour]."

A: "HR [X] · RR [X] · CRT [X] · SpO_2 [X]. Red flags: [list]. Given: [fluids/antibiotics]."

R: "Need urgent paediatric review and transfer."

Admit If	Discharge If
Red traffic light	Child drinking + passing urine
Amber + poor feeding or comorbidity	No red flags
Parent unable to cope	Parent understands safety-net
Safeguarding concerns	Follow-up arranged

Examiner Checklist

Assessment ✓	Management ✓
✓ ABCDE performed + verbalised	✓ Oxygen given if hypoxic
✓ NICE traffic light applied	✓ Fluid bolus 10 ml/kg (NOT 5)
✓ CRT checked + stated	✓ Antibiotics within 1 hour
✓ Full exposure (back + nappy area)	✓ IM benzylpenicillin if IV access difficult
✓ Glass test if rash	✓ Anaesthetics called for epiglottitis
✓ Immunisation status checked	✓ Senior involved early
✓ Wet nappies in last 24h asked	✓ Stop → Treat → Escalate → Reassess stated
✓ Safeguarding considered	✓ Two-layer safety-net given
✓ Parental concern acknowledged	✓ SBAR for handover

Station Recognition — One-Glance

Presentation	Flash	Urgency
Fever + well child, no focus	Green → safety-net	GREEN
Fever + lethargy + tachycardia	Sepsis until proven	RED
Fever + non-blanching rash + ill	RASH = meningococcal	RED
Fever + neck stiffness + photophobia	MENINGISM TRIAD	RED
Fever >5 days + rash + conjunctivitis	CRASH + BURN = Kawasaki	RED
Infant <3 months + any fever	<3 months = AUTOMATIC RED	RED
Fever without source	UTI until proven	AMBER
Fever + seizure	Febrile convulsion → simple vs complex	AMBER/RED

Final Exam Mantra

SICK RASH = all red flags · <3 months = URGENT · Non-blanching = IM benzylpenicillin NOW · 10 ml/kg NOT 5

Antibiotics within 1h · Epiglottitis = anaesthetics NOW, never examine throat

Bronchiolitis = O_2 if <92%, NO bronchodilators · Anaphylaxis = IM adrenaline 1:1000

Croup = dexamethasone + neb adrenaline if severe · Antipyretics = comfort only · Two-layer safety-net always

Gold Closing:

"Well or sick? Green, amber, or red? ABCDE performed, CRT checked, child fully undressed, glass test done, immunisations and wet nappies checked. Oxygen, 10 ml/kg fluids, antibiotics within 1 hour. IM benzylpenicillin if IV access difficult. Escalated via SBAR. Two-layer safety-net given. Antipyretics for comfort only. All doses checked with BNF for Children."

Non-blanching rash IM benzylpenicillin NOW	**10 ml/kg bolus** never 5 ml/kg	**Abx within 1 hour** every sepsis station	**<3 months fever** automatic red flag	**Epiglottitis** never examine throat
Bronchiolitis O_2 <92%, no bronchodilators	**Anaphylaxis** IM adrenaline 1:1000	**Antipyretics** comfort only, not prevention	**CRASH+BURN** Kawasaki if fever >5 days	**Two-layer safety-net** every discharge

TOP 5 EXAMINER Q&A · PAEDS I · FEBRILE CHILD & SEPSIS

Q1. What does the traffic-light system assess?	Colour, activity, respiratory status, hydration and other red flags to stratify febrile children into green, amber, red.
Q2. A non-blanching rash with fever means?	Meningococcal disease until proven otherwise: immediate IV/IM benzylpenicillin or ceftriaxone and emergency transfer.

TOP 5 EXAMINER Q&A · PAEDS I · FEBRILE CHILD & SEPSIS	
Q3. Which febrile infants need automatic full assessment?	Under 3 months with fever 38 or more: full septic screen and senior paediatric review.
Q4. What reassures you in a febrile child?	A child who smiles, plays, drinks and is consolable: behaviour outweighs the number on the thermometer.
Q5. Parental safety-netting for the green child?	Specific triggers to return: rash that does not fade, drowsiness, poor fluid intake, fewer wet nappies: written and verbal.
CURVEBALL	The "quiet, good baby" lying still during examination. Quietness in a febrile infant is a red flag, not a relief: escalate, do not be reassured.

CHAPTER 48 · PAEDS II: RESPIRATORY EMERGENCIES, CHOKING & FOREIGN BODY

SIGNS · FAST AIR · CEF · BAP · APS · C.A.L.M.

CORE · RED PATH · CAUTION — CRITICAL INSTANT FAIL RISK

Abbreviations used in this chapter: **APS** Antiphospholipid Syndrome

THINK — Core Rules:

Treatment FIRST, history SECOND in distressed child · Parental concern = severity marker · Position of comfort always

NEVER: Examine throat in epiglottitis · Blind finger sweep · Bronchodilators in bronchiolitis · Salbutamol alone for anaphylaxis

SAY — Golden Minute: "Using SIGNS and ABCDE. Allowing position of comfort. Treatment before detailed history. Reassessing after every intervention. Escalating immediately if SIGNS present."

SIGNS · FAST AIR · Scenario Clusters

SIGNS — Any ONE = escalate immediately:

S — Silent chest · I — Increased work of breathing · G — Gasping/apnoea · N — New altered consciousness · S — Saturations falling

FAST AIR: Feed/hydration · Airway patent? · SIGNS present? · Treatment started · Alert senior · Involve PICU · Reassess after every intervention

Clusters: CEF (upper) = Croup · Epiglottitis · Foreign body · BAP (lower) = Bronchiolitis · Asthma · Pneumonia · APS (systemic) = Anaphylaxis · Pertussis · Sepsis

Instant Fail Triggers

Examine throat in epiglottitis · Bronchodilators in bronchiolitis · Salbutamol instead of IM adrenaline for anaphylaxis

Blind finger sweep in choking · No escalation for SIGNS · Sending home unsafe child

Delay treatment to take history · Dismiss parental concern · No safety-netting

Normal CXR used to exclude foreign body — Normal CXR does NOT exclude FB. Refer for bronchoscopy if symptomatic.

CEF — Upper Airway: Croup · Epiglottitis · Foreign Body

Epiglottitis — DO NOT examine throat:

"Drooling + tripod position + toxic child = epiglottitis. DO NOT examine the throat — risk of complete airway obstruction."

1. DO NOT examine · 2. Call anaesthetics IMMEDIATELY · 3. Keep upright + calm with parent · 4. Minimal procedures · 5. Continuous SpO_2 monitoring

Croup — Bark + Stridor:

Mild: Oral dexamethasone → discharge + safety-net

Moderate: Oral dexamethasone · consider nebulised adrenaline · monitor

Severe: Nebulised adrenaline NOW + steroids · Admit · Monitor for REBOUND (effect temporary)

Impending failure: Call anaesthetics — manage as epiglottitis

Gestalt: "Bark + stridor = croup. Drooling + tripod = epiglottitis. If in doubt, treat as epiglottitis."

Choking + Foreign Body:

NEVER blind finger sweep — pushes object deeper · If unconscious → STOP manoeuvres → CPR immediately

Infant <1yr: 5 back blows (face down, head lower) + 5 chest thrusts. Alternate. NEVER abdominal thrusts.

Child >1yr: 5 back blows + 5 abdominal thrusts (Heimlich). Alternate.

Unilateral wheeze = inhaled FB until proven otherwise · Normal CXR does NOT exclude → bronchoscopy if symptomatic.

BAP — Lower Airway: Bronchiolitis · Asthma · Pneumonia

Bronchiolitis — NO bronchodilators:

NO salbutamol · NO ipratropium — not effective and harmful. Supportive: hydration · suction only if needed (not routine, NICE NG9) · O_2 if SpO_2 <92% · Monitor for APNOEA (highest risk <6 weeks / premature).

Severity	**Treatment**	**Escalate If**
Mild	Salbutamol via spacer (2–4 puffs). Steroids early.	No response to initial dose
Moderate	Salbutamol + ipratropium via spacer. Steroids. O_2 if hypoxic.	No response after 3 doses
Severe	Nebulised salbutamol + ipratropium. IV/IM magnesium. IV steroids.	Silent chest, exhaustion
Life-threatening	Silent chest + exhaustion + falling SpO_2	Call PICU/anaesthetics immediately

"Silent chest is pre-arrest — escalating to PICU and anaesthetics immediately."

Pneumonia vs Bronchiolitis:

Bronchiolitis: Infant <1yr · coryza · bilateral crackles/wheeze · NO antibiotics (supportive only)

Pneumonia: Child >2yrs · focal crackles · fever · lobar consolidation on CXR → antibiotics + senior review

APS — Systemic: Anaphylaxis · Pertussis · Sepsis

Anaphylaxis — IM adrenaline FIRST:
Rash + wheeze + hypotension + rapid onset = anaphylaxis. IM adrenaline immediately to anterolateral thigh. NOT salbutamol first.
Then: High-flow O_2 · IV fluids 10–20 ml/kg if hypotensive · call senior · observe for biphasic reaction up to 8h
Antihistamine + steroids: no longer routine in acute anaphylaxis (RCUK 2021); non-sedating oral antihistamine only after stabilisation, for skin symptoms

Condition	Actions
Pertussis	Paroxysmal cough + whoop + unvaccinated → Isolate immediately · Notify public health (notifiable disease) · Macrolide if early · Escalate if apnoea
Septic shock	Fever + toxic + poor perfusion → O_2 · blood cultures · IV/IO access · 20 ml/kg fluid bolus · IV antibiotics within 1 hour · PICU early. Note: 10 ml/kg is the initial bolus for sepsis without shock (see CH47); 20 ml/kg is for septic shock with poor perfusion. Reassess after every bolus and escalate to PICU early.

Spacer Technique — C.A.L.M.

C	Check device	Check spacer + inhaler · expiry dates · correct size
A	Assemble	Shake inhaler · insert into spacer · place mask over nose + mouth (no gaps)
L	Low/normal breath	Seal mask firmly · normal relaxed breathing — not forced inhalation
M	Medication	One puff · 5–10 normal breaths · wait 30 sec between puffs · rinse mouth after steroids

SAY — Parent Communication · Safety-Netting · Escalation

Empathy: "You did the right thing bringing them in. I can see this is frightening — we're acting quickly."
Parental concern: "I hear that you are worried — your concern is important information to me."
Two-layer safety-net:
Primary: "If breathing worsens or feeding drops, return immediately."
Emergency: "Rash that doesn't fade · stops drinking · drowsy · seizure → call 999 immediately."
After every intervention: "Reassessing ABCDE and SIGNS — [improved/no change/deteriorating]. Escalating if no improvement."

Examiner Checklist

Every Station ✓	Specific Scenarios ✓
✓ SIGNS mnemonic applied + verbalised	✓ Croup: steroids first + adrenaline if severe + rebound warned
✓ ABCDE performed	✓ Epiglottitis: throat NOT examined + anaesthetics called

Every Station ✓	Specific Scenarios ✓
✓ Position of comfort allowed	✓ Choking: age-specific manoeuvres + no finger sweep
✓ Treatment before detailed history	✓ Bronchiolitis: NO bronchodilators stated explicitly
✓ Parental concern acknowledged	✓ Asthma: silent chest = PICU called
✓ Reassessment after every intervention	✓ Anaphylaxis: IM adrenaline first — not salbutamol
✓ Escalation appropriate (PICU if SIGNS)	✓ Pertussis: isolated + public health notified
✓ Safety-net given (two-layer)	✓ Sepsis: O_2+cultures+fluids+abx+PICU within 1h

Scenario Quick Reference

Presentation	Diagnosis	Critical Action
Bark + stridor, 6m–3yrs	CROUP	Oral dexamethasone · neb adrenaline if severe
Drooling + tripod + toxic	EPIGLOTTITIS	DO NOT examine · call anaesthetics NOW
Sudden choking + coughing	FOREIGN BODY	Age manoeuvres · no finger sweep · CPR if unconscious
Wheeze + asthma history	ASTHMA	Salbutamol spacer · silent chest = PICU
Infant <1yr + coryza + wheeze	BRONCHIOLITIS	NO bronchodilators · O_2 if <92% · supportive
Rash + wheeze + hypotension	ANAPHYLAXIS	IM adrenaline 1:1000 immediately
Paroxysmal cough + whoop	PERTUSSIS	Isolate + notify public health
Toxic + poor perfusion + fever	SEPSIS	O_2 + cultures + 20ml/kg + abx within 1h + PICU

Final Exam Mantra

SIGNS: Silent · Increased work · Gasping · New altered consciousness · Sats falling → ANY ONE = escalate

CEF: Croup (bark+steroids±adrenaline) · Epiglottitis (drool+DO NOT examine+anaesthetics) · FB (manoeuvres, no sweep)

BAP: Bronchiolitis (NO bronchodilators) · Asthma (salbutamol, silent chest=PICU) · Pneumonia (antibiotics)

APS: Anaphylaxis (IM adrenaline first) · Pertussis (isolate+notify) · Sepsis (O_2+cultures+fluids+abx+PICU)

Always: position of comfort · reassess after every intervention · two-layer safety-net

SIGNS = escalate any one feature	No throat exam epiglottitis	Steroids croup not adrenaline alone	No bronchodilators bronchiolitis	IM adrenaline first anaphylaxis
No finger sweep choking always	Normal CXR does not exclude FB	Silent chest = PICU asthma pre-arrest	Pertussis isolate notify public health	Reassess always after every treatment

TOP 5 EXAMINER Q&A · PAEDS II · RESPIRATORY EMERGENCIES & CHOKING	
Q1. Croup vs epiglottitis at a glance?	Croup: barking cough, coryza, vaccinated child. Epiglottitis: drooling, toxic, sitting forward: no throat examination, airway team now.
Q2. Moderate croup treatment?	Oral dexamethasone 0.15 mg/kg single dose; nebulised adrenaline for severe cases with senior presence.
Q3. Bronchiolitis: what do parents need to know?	Supportive illness peaking day 3–5: feeding amount is the admission criterion: return if under half normal feeds, apnoeas or exhaustion.
Q4. Choking infant under 1: technique?	5 back blows then 5 chest thrusts (never abdominal thrusts in infants), alternating while help is called.
Q5. When does a wheezy child need admission?	Oxygen below 92%, poor response to bronchodilators, exhaustion, or social/safety-net concerns.
CURVEBALL	A toddler with sudden one-sided wheeze and no fever after playing with toys. Inhaled foreign body until excluded: this is bronchoscopy territory, not salbutamol territory.

CHAPTER 49 · PAEDS III: DEHYDRATION, GASTROENTERITIS & NEONATAL JAUNDICE

DEHYDRATE · DRIP · SOS · SHOCK · BILIOUS · SPLIT · PALE · JAUNDICE · KERNIC

CORE · CAUTION — INSTANT FAIL RISK · Paeds ED · GP · Neonatal Ward

Abbreviations used in this chapter: **CRT** Capillary Refill Time · **RUQ** Right Upper Quadrant

THINK — Core Rules:
Green vomit = obstruction until proven · Clinical signs > weight · ORS before IV unless shocked
Plot — do not guess · Conjugated = liver until proven · Pale stools = biliary atresia until proven
Unwell + jaundiced = sepsis until proven · When in doubt — ADMIT

SAY — Golden Rules: "Clinical signs > weight — I will NOT send a shocked child for weighing. Check glucose in every vomiting or lethargic child. Reassess after every intervention."

Instant Fail Triggers

Send shocked child for weight · Give IV fluids for mild dehydration · Call green vomit normal
Give phototherapy for conjugated jaundice · Discharge prolonged jaundice without split bilirubin
Miss pale stools without urgent referral · Not checking glucose · Guess phototherapy threshold

1. Dehydration Assessment — DEHYDRATE · DRIP · SUNNY

D	Dry mucous membranes / sunken eyes	Assess mouth + eyes
E	Eyes sunken / reduced urine	Sunken eyes = severe · ask about wet nappies (<6/24h = concern)
H	Heart rate ↑ / prolonged CRT	Tachycardia + CRT >3s = shock — do NOT wait for hypotension
Y	Young age / lethargy	Infants deteriorate faster — lower threshold
D	Decreased skin turgor / tenting	Tenting = moderate–severe
R	Red flags — BILIOUS mnemonic	Check all gastro/surgical red flags
A	Admission — SHOCK criteria	Any criterion = admit
T	Treatment: oral (SOS) vs IV (SHOCK)	Route based on clinical assessment
E	Escalate + reassess	After every intervention: HR, CRT, conscious level, urine

DRIP + Sunken Fontanelle: Dry mucous membranes · Reduced turgor · Irritability · Prolonged CRT (>3s) · Sunken fontanelle = SEVERE

Glucose: "Check capillary glucose in any vomiting or lethargic child — hypoglycaemia can mimic dehydration."

Sign	Mild (<5%)	Severe (>10%)
Skin turgor	Normal	Tenting
Conscious level	Irritable	Lethargic — DANGER
CRT	<2 sec	>3 sec — SHOCK
Fontanelle	Normal	Sunken
Heart rate	Normal	Tachycardia — EARLY sign
BP	Normal	Hypotension — LATE — do NOT wait
Urine	Normal	<6 wet nappies/24h

2. Rehydration — SOS · SHOCK · FLUID FAILS

SOS — Oral Route (give if all met)	SHOCK — IV Route (give if any met)
S — Stable (no shock, CRT <3s)	S — Shock (haemodynamic instability)
O — Orally willing (able to drink)	H — Haemodynamically unstable (tachy + CRT >3s)
S — Some dehydration (<10%)	O — Oral/NG challenge failed
	C — Conscious level reduced
	K — Ketoacidosis or >10% dehydration

ORS regimen: 5 ml every 2–3 minutes · if vomiting pause 10 min + restart · reassess at 4 hours · replace losses 1:1

NG before IV: If oral fails but child stable → NG ORS before IV fluids (preferred in paeds units)

IV bolus: 20 ml/kg 0.9% saline · reassess HR, CRT, conscious level, urine after EVERY bolus

FLUID FAILS — Pitfalls:

Fail to reassess after each bolus · Low-tonicity fluids given rapidly (hyponatraemia risk) · Underestimate severity · Ignore urine output · Delay fluids for blood tests

3. Gastroenteritis Red Flags — BILIOUS

BILIOUS — ANY ONE = ADMIT:

B — Bilious vomiting (green) = obstruction until proven — SURGICAL REVIEW NOW

I — Intractable pain · L — Lethargy · I — Intussusception signs (redcurrant jelly stool)

O — Oliguria (<6 wet nappies/24h) · U — Unable to tolerate oral · S — Stool blood

Intussusception triad: Colicky pain · redcurrant jelly stool · sausage-shaped mass (RUQ)
HUS (bloody diarrhoea): Pallor · oliguria · petechiae → Admit · FBC · U&Es · AVOID NSAIDs · AVOID antibiotics if E. coli O157 suspected

Vomiting Type	Likely Cause
Bilious (green)	Obstruction until proven — surgical emergency
Projectile (4–6 weeks)	Pyloric stenosis — palpable olive
Redcurrant jelly + mass	Intussusception
Bilious + unwell	Malrotation/volvulus — surgical emergency
Non-bilious + loose stools	Gastroenteritis

4. Neonatal Jaundice — JAUNDICE · SPLIT · PALE · KERNIC

	JAUNDICE History	Why It Matters
J	Jaundice onset	<24h = pathological — investigate immediately
A	Amount of feeding	Poor feeding worsens jaundice
U	Urine colour	Dark urine = conjugated until proven
N	Nappies	<6 wet/24h = concern
D	Dark urine?	Conjugated jaundice — liver disease
I	Infection signs	Sepsis risk — treat as sepsis if unwell
C	Colour of stools	Pale/chalky = biliary atresia until proven
E	Early gestation	Preterm = lower phototherapy threshold

SPLIT — Jaundice Workup:
S — Split bilirubin (conjugated >20% = pathological) · P — Plot on gestation-adjusted nomogram — NEVER guess
L — LFTs · I — Investigate if conjugated · T — Time >14d (term) / >21d (preterm) = prolonged → investigate
Phototherapy: UNCONJUGATED only. If conjugated >20% — do NOT start phototherapy — investigate cause.

Feature	Physiological	Pathological
Onset	>24 hours	<24 hours — INVESTIGATE
Duration	<14d term / <21d preterm	Prolonged — investigate
Conjugated	<20% of total	>20% = liver disease

Feature	Physiological	Pathological
Baby	Well	Unwell / poor feeding = sepsis screen

5. Biliary Atresia — PALE · Kernicterus — KERNIC

PALE — Biliary Atresia Red Flags:

P — Pale stools (white/chalky — use NHS stool colour card) · A — Alert baby (deceptively well-appearing)

L — Liver enlarged (hepatomegaly) · E — Early referral <8 WEEKS CRITICAL for Kasai procedure

SAY — Must-Say: "Pale stools + dark urine = biliary atresia until proven — urgent GI referral before 8 weeks. Outcomes worsen after 8 weeks."

KERNIC — Kernicterus Risk Factors:

K — Ketoacidosis/acidosis (displaces bilirubin) · E — Early gestation · R — Rapid rise · N — Neonatal sepsis · I — Immaturity · C — Conjugated? NO — kernicterus = UNCONJUGATED only

Signs of encephalopathy: Lethargy → irritability · poor feeding · high-pitched cry · opisthotonus · seizures → exchange transfusion

Examiner Checklist

Dehydration + Rehydration ✓	Jaundice ✓
✓ DEHYDRATE spine used	✓ JAUNDICE history mnemonic used
✓ CRT checked and stated	✓ Stool colour asked + NHS card offered
✓ Glucose checked (vomiting/lethargic)	✓ Urine colour asked
✓ Shocked child NOT sent for weighing	✓ SPLIT workup initiated
✓ SOS criteria checked before oral route	✓ Plotted on gestation-adjusted nomogram
✓ NG before IV if stable	✓ Conjugated >20% = no phototherapy
✓ 20ml/kg saline if shocked	✓ PALE checked (biliary atresia excluded)
✓ Reassessed after every bolus	✓ Referral <8 weeks if biliary atresia
✓ BILIOUS red flags checked	✓ KERNIC risk assessed
✓ Admit decision made	✓ Safety-net + follow-up arranged

Final Exam Mantra

Green vomit = obstruction · Clinical signs > weight · ORS before IV · NG before IV if stable · Check glucose always

Plot do not guess · Conjugated = liver · Pale stools = biliary atresia → refer <8 weeks

Phototherapy = unconjugated ONLY · KERNIC = unconjugated · Unwell + jaundiced = sepsis · When in doubt — ADMIT

Gold Closing:
"DEHYDRATE: CRT [X], signs [mild/severe], glucose checked. BILIOUS: [present/absent]. [SOS → ORS 5ml q2–3min / SHOCK → 20ml/kg saline, admitting]. Jaundice: SPLIT initiated, nomogram plotted, conjugated [<20%/≥20%], stool colour [yellow/pale], PALE checked, KERNIC risk assessed. Reassessing after every intervention. When in doubt — ADMIT."

Green vomit obstruction until proven	Clinical signs not weight in shock	Check glucose every vomiting/lethargic	ORS then NG then IV correct sequence	20ml/kg saline shocked child
BILIOUS = admit any one criterion	Plot do not guess nomogram always	Conjugated >20% no phototherapy	Pale stools refer <8 weeks	Kernic = unconjugated not conjugated

TOP 5 EXAMINER Q&A · PAEDS III · DEHYDRATION & NEONATAL JAUNDICE	
Q1. How do you assess dehydration severity?	Clinical signs: prolonged capillary refill, reduced skin turgor, sunken eyes, reduced urine output: shock is a separate category needing boluses.
Q2. First-line rehydration in gastroenteritis?	Oral rehydration solution little and often (or via NG tube): IV only for shock or ORS failure.
Q3. Bilious (green) vomiting in a neonate means?	Malrotation with volvulus until excluded: nil by mouth, NG tube, urgent surgical referral: never "observe".
Q4. Jaundice in the first 24 hours of life?	Always pathological: urgent serum bilirubin and haemolysis workup: never wait.
Q5. How is significant neonatal jaundice treated?	Plot bilirubin on the gestation-specific chart: phototherapy or exchange transfusion per thresholds: feed and hydrate.
CURVEBALL	Day-10 jaundice with pale stools and dark urine. Think biliary atresia: split bilirubin now: conjugated jaundice is a surgical clock that must not run out.

CHAPTER 50 · PAEDS IV: SEIZURES & FEBRILE CONVULSIONS

SEIZURE · FACTS · FEN · TRIGGERS · SAFE · Quiet Child Rule

CORE · GREEN PATH · CAUTION — CRITICAL INSTANT FAIL RISK

Abbreviations used in this chapter: **DVLA** Driver & Vehicle Licensing Agency · **EEG** Electroencephalogram · **HGV** Heavy Goods Vehicle · **PSV** Public Service Vehicle

THINK — Core Rules:

Seizure >5 minutes = rescue medication NOW · Buccal midazolam: between cheek and gum, NOT under tongue

Febrile convulsions do NOT cause brain damage · do NOT mean epilepsy — say BOTH explicitly

Recurrence risk = 30% (1 in 3) · most grow out by age 5 · Check glucose in EVERY seizure

Quiet + floppy + "not like them" = IMPENDING ARREST — escalate immediately

SAY — Golden Minute: "Is this child still seizing? I am timing from onset. If >5 minutes I give rescue medication. ABCDE, recovery position, blood glucose, FACTS check, meningitis signs. Reassure parents: not brain damage, not epilepsy, 30% recurrence."

SEIZURE — Master Framework

S	Still seizing? Time from onset	>5 min = rescue medication NOW
E	Evaluate ABCDE + recovery position	Recovery position if post-ictal
I	Identify trigger	Fever · head injury · check blood glucose
Z	Zero in on seizure type	Simple febrile vs complex vs first afebrile
U	Urgency — benzodiazepine by weight	Buccal midazolam: between cheek + gum
R	Reassure parents	Not brain damage · not epilepsy · 30% recurrence
E	Escalate + refer	FACTS red flags · FEN · meningitis pathway

Instant Fail Triggers

Not timing the seizure · Wrong benzodiazepine dose · Buccal midazolam under tongue (must be between cheek + gum)

No parental reassurance · Missing meningitis signs · No recurrence safety-net

Not referring first afebrile seizure · Forgetting blood glucose check

1. Benzodiazepine Ladder — Buccal Midazolam by Weight

Route: Between cheek and gum — NOT under tongue. Massage cheek gently after.

Weight	Buccal Midazolam Dose	Technique
<10 kg	2.5 mg	Between cheek + gum · massage cheek 30–60 sec

Weight	Buccal Midazolam Dose	Technique
10–20 kg	5 mg	Between cheek + gum · massage gently · both sides if needed
>20 kg	10 mg	Between cheek + gum · massage gently · monitor breathing

Step	Action
First dose (>5 min)	Buccal midazolam by weight — between cheek and gum
After 10 minutes	Repeat same dose ONCE if still seizing
After 2 doses (no response)	Call anaesthetics/PICU immediately — status epilepticus — IV therapy needed
If buccal not possible	Rectal diazepam — age-appropriate dose

Seizure duration thresholds:
>5 min: Rescue medication NOW · >15 min: Complex febrile — paediatric review · >30 min: Status epilepticus — anaesthetics/PICU

SAY — 2. Parental Reassurance — 8 Steps (Every Step = Marks)

1	"I can see this has been very frightening. You did exactly the right thing by coming in."
2	"Your child had a febrile convulsion. This happens when the temperature rises rapidly and temporarily lowers the seizure threshold."
3	"Febrile convulsions do NOT cause brain damage. They do NOT affect intelligence or development."
4	"This does NOT mean your child has epilepsy. Epilepsy is when someone has seizures without fever. This was triggered by the fever."
5	"About 1 in 3 children — 30% — will have another febrile convulsion with a future fever. Most children grow out of them by age 5."
6	SAFE instructions — give all 4 steps (see below)
7	"Treat the fever with paracetamol or ibuprofen — but treating fever does NOT prevent febrile convulsions."
8	**Safety-net:** "Return if: seizure >5 min · another seizure · not waking normally within 1 hour · you are worried."

SAFE Instructions:
S — Stay calm + time the seizure · A — Alert 999 if >5 minutes · F — First aid: recovery position, nothing in mouth · E — Exact details: record duration + type

3. FACTS Red Flags · Meningitis Check

	FACTS — ANY ONE = Complex → Paediatric Review	**Action**
F	Focal features (one limb, eye deviation, Todd's paresis)	Urgent paediatric review · consider EEG + neuroimaging
A	Age <6 months	Higher risk · senior review · sepsis workup
C	Chronic duration >15 minutes	Paediatric review
T	Two+ seizures in 24 hours	Paediatric review · investigate cause
S	Signs of meningitis / Still not baseline at 1h	Sepsis pathway + IV abx if meningitis · Senior review if not baseline

> Meningitis — Always Check in Fever + Seizure:
> Neck stiffness → sepsis pathway · Non-blanching rash → IV antibiotics IMMEDIATELY · Bulging fontanelle → urgent senior review
> **Infant signs:** Irritability · high-pitched cry · poor feeding · lethargy · bulging fontanelle

Simple vs Complex Febrile Convulsion

Feature	**Simple**	**Complex**
Age	6 months to 5 years	Any — but <6 months = higher risk
Type	Generalised tonic-clonic	Focal features
Duration	<15 minutes	>15 minutes
Frequency	Single in 24 hours	Two or more in 24 hours
Recovery	Baseline within 1 hour	Not baseline at 1 hour
Action	Reassure + SAFE + safety-net	Urgent paediatric review

THINK — 4. FEN · TRIGGERS · Quiet Child Rule

> **FEN — First Afebrile Seizure:**
> F — First seizure → urgent paediatric referral · E — EEG within 2 weeks · N — Neuroimaging (MRI if focal or <1yr; urgent CT if post-traumatic)
> Also: ABCDE · blood glucose · home safety advice (no unsupervised bathing, heights)

	TRIGGERS — Breakthrough Epilepsy	**Ask This**
T	Treatment compliance	"Taking medication every day without missing doses?"
R	Recent illness	"Any fever or infection recently?"
I	Inadequate sleep	"Any missed sleep or long journeys?"
G	Growth/weight change	"Have they grown significantly? Dose may need adjusting."

	TRIGGERS — Breakthrough Epilepsy	Ask This
G	Generic switches	"Any change in brand or different pharmacy?"
E	Emotional stress	"Any stress at home or school?"
R	Rash/side effects	"Any rash, drowsiness, or behaviour changes?"

Quiet Child Rule — IMPENDING ARREST:
"Quiet + floppy + drowsy + stops fighting + parent says not like them = impending arrest — escalate immediately."
"A quiet child is a dying child."

Examiner Checklist

Management ✓	Communication ✓
✓ Seizure timed from onset	✓ Fear acknowledged first
✓ ABCDE + recovery position	✓ Mechanism explained (fever + rapid rise)
✓ Blood glucose checked	✓ NOT brain damage — stated explicitly
✓ Buccal midazolam: correct weight dose	✓ NOT epilepsy — stated explicitly
✓ Between cheek + gum stated	✓ 30% recurrence + grows out by age 5
✓ Repeat dose after 10 min if seizing	✓ SAFE instructions — all 4 steps given
✓ Anaesthetics/PICU if 2 doses fail	✓ Fever treatment (does not prevent)
✓ FACTS: all 5 checked	✓ Safety-net: all 4 return criteria
✓ Meningitis: neck/rash/fontanelle	✓ Quiet child escalated if seen
✓ FEN referral if first afebrile	✓ Follow-up arranged

Final Exam Mantra

Time it → >5 min = rescue med NOW · Buccal midazolam: cheek+gum, by weight · Repeat once at 10 min · 2 doses fail = anaesthetics

FACTS: Focal · Age <6m · Chronic >15min · Two+ · Signs meningitis = ANY ONE → paed review

Parent script: NOT brain damage · NOT epilepsy · 30% recurrence · SAFE · fever Tx not preventative

FEN: refer + EEG + neuroimaging · TRIGGERS: 7 questions · Quiet child = impending arrest

Gold Closing:

"SEIZURE applied. [Simple febrile:] FACTS negative, baseline within 1 hour. Parental reassurance: not brain damage, not epilepsy, 30% recurrence. SAFE instructions given. [If complex:] FACTS positive — paediatric review. [If >5 min:] Buccal midazolam by weight, between cheek and gum. [If status:] Anaesthetics/PICU called. Blood glucose checked. Safety-net: return if >5 min, another seizure, not waking, or worried."

>5 min = rescue med buccal midazolam NOW	Cheek + gum NOT under tongue	<10kg = 2.5mg 10-20kg = 5mg, >20kg = 10mg	FACTS = paed review any one criterion	Not brain damage say explicitly
Not epilepsy say explicitly	30% recurrence grows out by age 5	SAFE instructions all 4 steps	Check glucose every seizure	Quiet child impending arrest

DVLA Advice — Seizures

Group 1 (car/motorcycle): First unprovoked seizure: 6 months off driving (12 months if investigations show increased risk). Established epilepsy: 12 months seizure-free required. Medication withdrawal: stop driving during the change and for 6 months after. Sleep-only seizures may permit driving if an established asleep-only pattern. Specialist advice required in all cases.

Group 2 (HGV/PSV): Stricter long-term restrictions — specialist advice required. Notify DVLA in all seizure cases.

CAUTION — Must-Say: "You must stop driving and inform the DVLA. I will document this advice clearly today."

TOP 5 EXAMINER Q&A · PAEDS IV · SEIZURES & FEBRILE CONVULSIONS	
Q1. Define a simple febrile convulsion.	Generalised tonic-clonic seizure under 15 minutes, once in 24 hours, in a febrile child aged 6 months to 5 years, with full recovery.
Q2. What do parents need after a first simple febrile convulsion?	Reassurance about benign prognosis, recovery-position first aid, when to call 999 (over 5 minutes), and that antipyretics do not prevent recurrence.
Q3. When does a febrile seizure need admission?	Complex features, first seizure under 18 months, incomplete recovery, no clear focus, or parental inability to cope.
Q4. Status epilepticus in a child: first drug?	At 5 minutes: IV lorazepam, or buccal midazolam without access: repeat once, then escalate to second line.
Q5. What must you always check during any childhood seizure?	Glucose: and after it, ask about the quiet drowsy child who is "just postictal": reassess.
CURVEBALL	Parents filmed the episode on a phone. Watch it: home video is often the single most useful diagnostic tool you will get: praise them for it.

CHAPTER 51 · PAEDS V: SAFEGUARDING & NON-ACCIDENTAL INJURY

HISTORY · TEN-4-FACES-P · FACES · HEADS · MIMIC · FABRICATE · CHILD · REFER · ADMIT · SAFE

CORE · CAUTION — INSTANT FAIL RISK · Paeds ED · GP · Safeguarding

Abbreviations used in this chapter: **AHT** Abusive Head Trauma · **FII** Fabricated or Induced Illness · **ITP** Immune Thrombocytopenia · **NAI** Non-Accidental Injury

DISTINCTION — Golden Triad of Fail — Missing ANY = very high risk of failing:
1. Missing bruising in a non-mobile infant · 2. Accepting inconsistent history without escalation · 3. Discharging without senior review + safeguarding
"Those who don't cruise, don't bruise" — ANY bruising in non-mobile infant = red flag
Posterior rib + metaphyseal corner fractures = HIGHLY SPECIFIC for NAI · Retinal haemorrhage → ophthalmology within 24h
Legal duty: Can share information without parental consent if child is at risk of significant harm

SAY — Golden Minute: "This history is inconsistent with the injury pattern — I have a safeguarding concern. I am fully undressing the child. Using TEN-4-FACES-P, HISTORY, and FACES. Escalating to senior now. Not discharging without safeguarding plan."

Instant Fail Triggers

Miss bruising in non-mobile infant · Accept inconsistent history · Challenge parent alone
Not examine entire body · Estimate bruise age by colour · Miss posterior rib / metaphyseal fractures
No ophthalmology within 24h for retinal haemorrhage · Discharge without safeguarding · Accuse parent directly

1. History Red Flags — HISTORY Mnemonic

H	History changes	Different versions from parents · changes at second telling
I	Inconsistent with injury	"Rolled off sofa" → spiral femur in 3-month-old = not compatible
S	Stimulus absent	No trauma explanation — "he just started crying"
T	Timing unclear / delay	Significant delay between alleged injury and presentation
O	Other injuries	Old injuries on exam or imaging · multiple healing stages
R	Repeated presentations	Multiple ED attendances or different hospitals
Y	Young age (<1 year)	Infants most vulnerable — cannot protect themselves

Safe challenge: "I'm a little confused — can you help me understand how this happened?" · Never challenge parent alone · Involve senior first

Document verbatim: "Mother said: 'He just fell off the sofa'" — in quotation marks with time, date, who was present

2. Bruising — TEN-4-FACES-P + Cruising Rule

"Those who don't cruise, don't bruise" — ANY bruising in a non-mobile infant = highly concerning for NAI.

	TEN-4-FACES-P Location	NAI Significance
T	Torso (chest, abdomen, back)	Protected areas — not areas of accidental impact
E	Ears (pinna, behind ears)	Almost never accidental
N	Neck	Highly suspicious — consider grip/strangulation
4	4 years and under (any infant <4 months: ALL suspicious)	Cannot cause own bruising
F	Frenulum (torn)	Sentinel injury — predictor of future severe harm
A	Angle of jaw	Grip marks from shaking
C	Cheek (slap marks)	Patterned — deliberate force
E	Eyelids	Consider AHT — arrange ophthalmology
S	Subconjunctival haemorrhage	Arrange ophthalmology — retinal haemorrhage screen
P	Pre-mobile infant — ANY bruising	External force required — automatic red flag

Never estimate bruise age by colour — unreliable and must never appear in documentation.

Sentinel injuries: Torn frenulum · bruise in non-mobile infant — small injuries predicting future severe harm

3. Fractures — FACES · Abusive Head Trauma — HEADS

	FACES Fracture	NAI Significance	Action
F	Femur spiral (non-mobile infant)	Cannot create rotational force by falling	Skeletal survey + safeguarding
A	Angular (metaphyseal corner)	HIGHLY SPECIFIC for NAI — violent pulling/twisting	Urgent safeguarding + skeletal survey

	FACES Fracture	NAI Significance	Action
C	Costal (posterior rib)	HIGHLY SPECIFIC — AP chest squeeze during shaking	Skeletal survey + ophthalmology + safeguarding
E	Epiphyseal separation	Rare accidental — pulling/twisting	Senior review + skeletal survey
S	Skull (complex/depressed)	Complex more suspicious than simple linear	CT head + senior + safeguarding

HEADS — Abusive Head Trauma:
H — Head injury signs · E — Eyes: retinal haemorrhage → ophthalmology WITHIN 24h · A — Apnoea · D — Developmental regression · S — Subdural haemorrhage
Shaken baby triad: Retinal haemorrhage (bilateral, multi-layered, to periphery) + Subdural + Encephalopathy

4. Medical Mimics — MIMIC · FII — FABRICATE · Neglect

MIMIC — Consider but do not delay escalation:
M — Mongolian spots (present from birth, grey-blue, buttocks) · I — Inherited bleeding (ITP/haemophilia → clotting screen)
M — Metabolic bone (OI: blue sclera, recurrent fractures) · I — Infections · C — Cultural practices (coining/cupping)

FABRICATE — Fabricated or Induced Illness (FII):
Frequent attendances · Alleged not witnessed · By proxy · Results normal · Inconsistent · Carer calm · Avoids reassurance · Treatment escalations · Exaggeration

Neglect types: Physical (poor hygiene, FTT) · Medical (missed appointments) · Supervisory (child left alone) · Emotional (frozen watchfulness)

5. Documentation (CHILD) · Communication · Escalation (REFER)

C	Clear verbatim history	Quote parents EXACTLY in quotation marks with time, date, who present
H	Head-to-toe examination	Fully undress · chaperone for genital/perianal exam · all skin surfaces
I	Imaging	Skeletal survey <2yr · CT head if AHT · repeat skeletal survey 10–14 days
L	Liaise with seniors	Document who informed, when, and their response
D	Document with body maps	Injuries: measure (cm) · describe shape · do NOT estimate age by colour

Say to parents: "I'm concerned about these injuries. This is routine — we do this for any child with injuries like this. My priority is the child's safety."
Never say: "I think you hurt your child" · "Social services will take your child away" · Estimate bruise age · Challenge alone

REFER — Escalation Steps:
R — Recognise red flags · E — Escalate to senior immediately · F — Formal safeguarding referral · E — Explain to parents · R — Review + siblings assessed
Legal duty: "I can share information without parental consent if child is at risk of significant harm."
Do NOT leave child alone with caregiver during assessment.

Investigations · ADMIT · SAFE Discharge

Investigation	Indication
Skeletal survey	All children <2yr with suspected NAI · Repeat at 10–14 days for healing fractures
CT head	Head injury · neurological signs · any infant with suspected NAI
Ophthalmology <24h	ANY suspected AHT — dilated retinal exam by paediatric ophthalmologist
FBC + clotting screen	All suspected NAI — exclude ITP, haemophilia, Von Willebrand
LFTs + amylase	Suspected abdominal injury — solid organ damage often clinically silent

ADMIT — Any ONE = admit: Any bruising in non-mobile infant · Dangerous fracture · Multiple injuries · Inconsistent history · TEN-4-FACES-P distribution
SAFE discharge — ALL FOUR must be confirmed: Safeguarding team agrees · All investigations done · Family assessed · Environment safe
Siblings: Risk applies to all children in household — safeguarding team must assess all siblings

Examiner Checklist

Recognition + Examination ✓	Escalation + Documentation ✓
✓ HISTORY red flags identified	✓ Senior involved immediately
✓ History inconsistency flagged	✓ Formal safeguarding referral made
✓ Verbatim history in quotation marks	✓ Child not left alone with caregiver
✓ Child fully undressed	✓ All siblings identified + safeguarded
✓ Chaperone for genital/perianal exam	✓ Legal duty stated (share without consent)
✓ TEN-4-FACES-P applied	✓ Communication non-accusatory
✓ Cruising rule stated	✓ CHILD documentation completed
✓ Bruise age NOT estimated by colour	✓ Body maps used
✓ FACES fractures assessed	✓ ADMIT criteria checked
✓ HEADS + ophthalmology <24h	✓ SAFE discharge criteria confirmed

Recognition + Examination ✓	Escalation + Documentation ✓
✓ MIMIC considered + clotting screen	✓ FABRICATE considered if appropriate

Final Exam Mantra

Golden Triad of Fail: Miss bruising non-mobile · Accept inconsistent history · Discharge without safeguarding

"Those who don't cruise, don't bruise" · Post rib + metaphyseal = HIGHLY SPECIFIC · Ophthalmology within 24h

CHILD: verbatim + body maps · REFER: escalate + senior + formal referral · Never accuse parent directly

Legal duty: share without parental consent if risk · SAFE: all 4 criteria before discharge · Siblings always

Gold Closing:

"HISTORY inconsistency identified. TEN-4-FACES-P: bruising on torso in non-mobile infant — red flag. FACES: posterior rib fracture — highly specific for NAI — skeletal survey arranged. HEADS: ophthalmology within 24h. MIMIC: clotting screen arranged. CHILD documentation: verbatim, body maps. REFER: senior informed, formal safeguarding referral. SAFE: will not discharge without all 4 criteria. Siblings assessed. Legal duty stated."

"Don't cruise, don't bruise" non-mobile = red flag	TEN-4-FACES-P bruising distribution	Post rib + metaphyseal highly specific NAI	Ophthalmology <24h retinal haemorrhage	Never estimate bruise age by colour unreliable
CHILD documentation verbatim + body maps	REFER escalation senior now	Legal duty share without consent	SAFE discharge all 4 criteria	Siblings always household risk

TOP 5 EXAMINER Q&A · PAEDS V · SAFEGUARDING & NON-ACCIDENTAL INJURY

Q1. What is the TEN-4 rule?	Bruising on Torso, Ears or Neck in under-4s, or any bruise in under-4-months: red flags for abuse.
Q2. Which fracture patterns raise concern?	Metaphyseal corner fractures, posterior rib fractures, fractures in non-mobile infants, and multiple fractures of different ages.
Q3. A story that does not fit the injury: what next?	Document verbatim, examine fully, senior paediatric review, safeguarding referral: the child does not go home until safe.
Q4. Mimics you must exclude?	Coagulation disorders, osteogenesis imperfecta, Mongolian blue spots, coining/cupping practices: investigate while safeguarding proceeds.
Q5. How do you talk to parents during a safeguarding workup?	Honest and non-accusatory: "our duty is to check every possible cause, including injury": hostility helps no one, least of all the child.
CURVEBALL	The parent wants to take the non-mobile bruised infant home "against advice". The child's safety overrides: senior, safeguarding team and if necessary police protection: this is the one discharge you never allow.

CHAPTER 52 · PAEDS VI: PAEDIATRIC ASSESSMENT TOOLKIT & ADOLESCENT HEALTH

PAT · TICLS · PEWS · HEADSS · FIRM · RAISE · SPOT · Quiet Child Rule

CORE · YELLOW PATH · GREEN PATH · CAUTION — CRITICAL INSTANT FAIL RISK

Abbreviations used in this chapter: **AVPU** Alert, Voice, Pain, Unresponsive · **CRT** Capillary Refill Time · **NAI** Non-Accidental Injury

THINK — First Question: "How sick is this child? Stable or unstable? Do I need help now?"
Instant Fail Triggers: Missing non-blanching rash · Quiet Child not escalated · Promising secrecy to child · Breaking confidentiality without explaining · Not assessing Fraser competence · Measles not notified

SAY — Golden Rule: "How sick? Stable/unstable? PAT + TICLS first. Quiet = floppy = impending arrest = CALL HELP. Non-blanching rash + fever = sepsis NOW. Confidentiality before HEADSS. SPOT always. If uncertain — ADMIT."

1. First Impression — PAT · TICLS · PEWS · Quiet Child Rule

PAT — Paediatric Assessment Triangle (10-second check):
Appearance (TICLS) · Work of breathing (recession, grunting, rate) · Circulation to skin (colour, CRT, mottling)
ANY red flag → UNSTABLE → call for help immediately

TICLS: T — Tone · I — Interaction · C — Consolability · L — Look/Gaze · S — Speech/Cry
PEWS (concept only): Behaviour (irritable/lethargic?) · Cardiovascular (colour, CRT) · Respiratory (rate, recession, grunting, silent chest). If concerning → escalate immediately.

QUIET CHILD RULE — IMPENDING ARREST:
Stops crying · stops fighting · floppy · drowsy · parent says "not like them" = ESCALATE IMMEDIATELY

	ABCDE	Red Flags
A	Airway — patent? stridor? silent?	Stridor · drooling · silence
B	Breathing — rate, recession, grunting, sats	Tachypnoea · recession · grunting · apnoea
C	Circulation — HR, CRT, colour	Tachycardia · prolonged CRT · mottling
D	Disability — AVPU, glucose	Decreasing AVPU · hypoglycaemia

	ABCDE	Red Flags
E	Exposure — rash, fever, injuries	Non-blanching rash · unexplained bruising

Always check: Pain (FLACC/Faces/0–10) · Hydration (urine output, CRT, feeding) · Immunisation status · Growth/development

2. Fever Red Flags · Rash Recognition

Rash	Key Feature	Action
Meningococcal	Non-blanching · petechial/purpuric + fever	SEPSIS PATHWAY immediately
Chickenpox	'Dew drop on rose petal' · vesicular · centripetal	Isolate · NO ibuprofen · NO aspirin · exclude until vesicles crusted
Scarlet fever	Sandpaper-like + strawberry tongue	Antibiotics · notify public health · exclude 24h after treatment starts
Measles	Maculopapular + coryza + conjunctivitis · head → down	NOTIFIABLE — isolate + notify public health IMMEDIATELY

Chickenpox: NO ibuprofen (necrotising fasciitis risk) · NO aspirin (Reye's syndrome)
Measles: NOTIFY PUBLIC HEALTH — legal requirement. Isolate — airborne precautions.
Infection control: Any rash + fever → PPE. Epiglottitis: DO NOT examine throat. NAI: avoid repeated exams.

3. Adolescent Health — Confidentiality · HEADSS · FIRM · RAISE

Step 0 — Confidentiality FIRST (before HEADSS):
"Before we start: everything we discuss is confidential unless I'm worried you or someone else is at serious risk of harm. If that happens, I will always explain first. Is that okay?"
"I'd like to speak with you alone for a few minutes — Parent, would you mind waiting outside?"

H	Home	"Who lives at home? How do you get along?"
E	Education/Employment	"School? How are things going?"
A	Activities	"What do you do for fun? Friends?"
D	Drugs	"Do friends smoke, vape, drink? Have you tried anything?"
D	Diet/Eating	"Any concerns about weight or body image?"
S	Sexuality	"Are you in a relationship? Questions about sex or contraception?"
S	Safety/Suicide	"Have you felt so sad you wanted to hurt yourself? Do you feel safe at home?"

Under-13 rule: Sexual activity = AUTOMATIC safeguarding referral — child protection
13–15: Assess coercion · grooming · power imbalance → safeguarding if concerns

FIRM — Gillick/Fraser Competence (under-16):
F — Fully understands advice + implications · I — In best interests · R — Risks understood · M — Mature + voluntary (free from coercion)
All 4 YES → proceed without parental consent. Any NO → safeguarding + consider parental involvement. Document verbatim.

RAISE — When to break confidentiality:
R — Risk to self · A — Abuse disclosed · I — Illegal activity with harm · S — Safeguarding · E — Exploitation (grooming, County Lines)

4. Safeguarding — SPOT · Admission · Public Health

SPOT — Safeguarding Mnemonic:
S — Stories inconsistent · P — Parent behaviour concerning · O — Observations worrying · T — Trauma unexplained
If disclosure: Listen without interrupting · Do NOT promise secrecy · Document verbatim · Escalate immediately

Admit If	**Notifiable Diseases**
PEWS high or red flag	Measles — NOTIFY IMMEDIATELY + isolate
Toxic appearance	Scarlet fever (outbreaks) — notify
Dehydration moderate/severe	Pertussis — notify
Safeguarding concerns	Mumps / Rubella — notify
Parental unable to cope	Chickenpox in pregnancy — notify
UNCERTAINTY → ADMIT	Always better safe than sorry

Examiner Checklist

Assessment + Rashes ✓	**Adolescent + Safeguarding ✓**
✓ First impression triad assessed	✓ Confidentiality statement delivered FIRST
✓ PAT + TICLS applied	✓ Offered to speak alone
✓ Unstable child escalated	✓ HEADSS domains covered
✓ Quiet Child Rule considered	✓ Under-13 rule known + applied
✓ ABCDE performed	✓ FIRM assessed if under-16
✓ Pain + hydration + immunisations	✓ RAISE — breaks confidentiality if needed
✓ Non-blanching rash → sepsis	✓ SPOT applied throughout
✓ Chickenpox: no ibuprofen	✓ Disclosure: no secrecy + escalate

Assessment + Rashes ✓	Adolescent + Safeguarding ✓
✓ Measles: notified + isolated	✓ Admission criteria considered
✓ Parental concern as severity marker	✓ If uncertain → ADMIT stated

Final Exam Mantra

How sick? → PAT + TICLS → Stable/unstable → PEWS → ABCDE (pain, hydration, immunisations)
Fever flags → Rashes: non-blanching=sepsis · vesicular=chickenpox(no ibuprofen) · sandpaper=scarlet fever · maculopapular=measles(NOTIFY+isolate)
Quiet Child = impending arrest · Adolescent: confidentiality FIRST + alone + HEADSS + FIRM · Under-13 = safeguarding
RAISE to break confidentiality · SPOT safeguarding always · If uncertain — ADMIT

Gold Closing:
"PAT + TICLS performed. Child is [stable/unstable]. ABCDE done: pain assessed, hydration checked, immunisations. Fever red flags checked — [rash identified and acted on]. Quiet Child Rule considered. [If adolescent:] Confidentiality explained first, spoke alone, HEADSS completed, FIRM assessed. SPOT applied throughout. Disposition: [admit/discharge]. If uncertain — admit. Safety-net given. Documented."

PAT + TICLS first impression always	Quiet child impending arrest	Non-blanching rash sepsis pathway NOW	Chickenpox no ibuprofen, no aspirin	Measles notify + isolate legal
Confidentiality first before HEADSS	Under-13 sex automatic safeguarding	FIRM = Fraser all 4 criteria	SPOT always safeguarding screen	If uncertain ADMIT

TOP 5 EXAMINER Q&A · PAEDS VI · ASSESSMENT TOOLKIT & ADOLESCENT HEALTH

Q1. What is the Paediatric Assessment Triangle?	Appearance, work of breathing, circulation to skin: a 30-second doorway impression that triages sick from not-sick.
Q2. What does PEWS add?	Age-adjusted early warning scoring that triggers structured escalation: state the score and the action.
Q3. What is HEADSS for?	Adolescent psychosocial screen: Home, Education, Activities, Drugs, Sexuality, Suicide/mood: ask alone, confidentially.
Q4. How do you handle adolescent confidentiality?	Confidential unless safety requires sharing: say so up front: competent teens can consent to treatment.
Q5. Examining an adolescent: what is good practice?	Offer a chaperone, examine with consent and privacy, and involve them: not just the parent: in every decision.
CURVEBALL	Mum answers every question for her 15-year-old. Create separation naturally: "I always speak with young people alone for part of the visit": that is where the real history lives.

CHAPTER 53 · PAEDS VII: CHILDHOOD VACCINATION & VACCINE HESITANCY

SAFER · VACCINE · UK Schedule 2026 · Herd Immunity · Contraindications · Catch-Up

VERY HIGH · GREEN PATH · CAUTION — MODERATE INSTANT FAIL RISK

Abbreviations used in this chapter: **HPV** Human Papillomavirus · **MMR** Measles, Mumps & Rubella · **PCV** Packed Cell Volume

THINK — Core Rules:
Never argue with vaccine-hesitant parent · SAFER for MMR concerns · Wakefield retracted 2010 — no link proven
95% herd immunity threshold · Shared decision — not coercion · Escalate if refuses all
Instant Fail Triggers: Arguing with parent · Forgetting contraindications · Cannot explain herd immunity · No shared decision-making · Can't explain Wakefield retraction

SAY — Golden Minute: "Routine, catch-up, or hesitant? SAFER for MMR. VACCINE for hesitancy. Wakefield retracted 2010. 95% herd immunity. Shared decision — not coercion."

UK Vaccination Schedule 2026

Age	Vaccines	Key
8 weeks	6-in-1 · PCV · Rotavirus (oral) · MenB	6-in-1 = Diphtheria, Tetanus, Pertussis, Polio, Hib, Hep B
12 weeks	6-in-1 (2nd) · Rotavirus (2nd)	
16 weeks	6-in-1 (3rd) · PCV (2nd) · MenB (2nd)	
1 year	MMR (1st) · PCV (3rd) · MenB (3rd) · Hib/MenC	MMR 1st dose
2–8 years	Flu (annual)	
3 years 4 months	MMR (2nd) · 4-in-1 pre-school booster	MMR 2nd dose
12–13 years	HPV (2 doses)	Human papillomavirus
14 years	3-in-1 (Td/IPV) · MenACWY	

Contraindications — RED LIGHTS vs GREEN LIGHTS

✗ TRUE Contraindications — Do NOT vaccinate	✓ NOT Contraindications — Vaccinate
Anaphylaxis to previous dose or component	Mild illness without fever
Severe immunosuppression (chemo, high-dose steroids) — LIVE vaccines	Egg allergy (non-anaphylaxis) — MMR is SAFE
Pregnancy — live vaccines (MMR, varicella)	Family history of autism or seizures

✗ TRUE Contraindications — Do NOT vaccinate	✓ NOT Contraindications — Vaccinate
	Asthma, eczema, prematurity
	Breastfeeding · antibiotic use
	Prematurity — vaccinate at CHRONOLOGICAL age

MMR Counselling — SAFER · Herd Immunity · The Autism Myth

S	Sit and listen	"Tell me what concerns you have about the MMR vaccine."
A	Acknowledge concerns	"I understand why you might be worried — there's a lot of information online."
F	Facts, not opinions	"The Wakefield paper was retracted in 2010. He was struck off. Multiple large studies show no link."
E	Explain benefits	"Measles can cause pneumonia, encephalitis, and death. Before the vaccine, hundreds died each year."
R	Reassure + return	"Take this leaflet home. Come back when ready — no pressure."

Wakefield Myth — Key Facts:
Paper based on 12 children · Data fabricated · Retracted 2010 · GMC struck Wakefield off for serious professional misconduct
Multiple large studies — millions of children — no link between MMR and autism
Autism timing: "Autism is often diagnosed around the same age MMR is given — this is coincidence, NOT causation."

Herd Immunity Script:
"When enough people are vaccinated, the disease can't spread — this protects those who can't be vaccinated, like newborns or children on chemotherapy. We need 95% coverage. When rates drop below this, we see outbreaks."

Vaccine Hesitancy — VACCINE Mnemonic · Catch-Up

V	Validate concerns	"It's completely understandable to have questions about vaccination."
A	Ask open questions	"What have you heard? What worries you most?"
C	Clarify misinformation	"Let me explain what the evidence actually shows."
C	Check understanding	"Does that make sense? What are your thoughts now?"
I	Invite questions	"What else would you like to know?"
N	Negotiate next steps	"Would you like more information? Shall we meet again?"
E	Empower decision	"This is your decision — we're here to support you."

Catch-Up — Golden Rule: "Any missed vaccine can be given at any age. It's never too late to get protected."
6-in-1 doses: give remaining at monthly intervals · MMR both doses missed: give both, 3 months apart · Pre-school booster: give if missed up to 10 years

Escalate to senior if: Parent refuses all vaccines despite discussion · Complex medical history · Safeguarding concerns · Accelerated schedule requested
SBAR: "S: Hesitant parent re MMR. B: Wakefield explained. A: Uncertain, wants time. R: Would you like to speak with her?"

Examiner Checklist

Knowledge + Safety ✓	**Communication ✓**
✓ UK schedule known (8w/12w/16w/1y/3y4m/12-13/14)	✓ Opened with open questions
✓ 8-week vaccines: 6-in-1 + PCV + Rota + MenB	✓ Concerns validated non-judgmentally
✓ MMR: 1st at 1 year, 2nd at 3y4m	✓ SAFER applied for MMR
✓ TRUE contraindications ruled out	✓ Wakefield retraction explained
✓ Egg allergy = NOT contraindication stated	✓ Autism coincidence/causation explained
✓ Prematurity = chronological age	✓ Herd immunity explained with 95%
✓ Catch-up plan offered	✓ Shared decision-making demonstrated
✓ Senior escalation if refusal	✓ Written information offered
✓ Documentation mentioned	✓ Safety-net given

Final Exam Mantra

Routine/catch-up/hesitant? · SAFER for MMR · VACCINE for hesitancy · 95% herd immunity
Wakefield retracted 2010 · no link proven · autism = coincidence not causation
RED LIGHTS: anaphylaxis + severe immunosuppression · GREEN LIGHTS: mild illness + egg allergy + family history
Catch-up any age any time · Never argue · Shared decision · Escalate if refuses all

Gold Closing:
"I've listened to your concerns, explained the evidence — including that the MMR-autism link has been completely disproven — and discussed herd immunity. Contraindications checked. [If vaccinating:] Going ahead with routine vaccines now, written info given. [If deferring:] Take the leaflet, discuss with your partner, come back when ready. This has been a shared decision. Documentation completed."

8-week vaccines 6-in-1+PCV+Rota+MenB	MMR 1st dose 1 year	MMR 2nd dose 3 years 4 months	95% herd immunity protects vulnerable	Wakefield retracted 2010 GMC struck off
Egg allergy = safe not a contraindication	SAFER mnemonic MMR counselling	VACCINE mnemonic hesitancy approach	Catch-up any age it's never too late	Escalate if refuses all senior + document

TOP 5 EXAMINER Q&A · PAEDS VII · CHILDHOOD VACCINATION	
Q1. Parent says vaccines cause autism. Your response?	Acknowledge the worry, state clearly the claim was fraudulent and disproven by massive studies, and pivot to their specific concerns.
Q2. What is herd immunity and why explain it?	High community coverage protects those who cannot be vaccinated: it reframes vaccination as protecting others too.
Q3. Which are true contraindications?	Anaphylaxis to a previous dose or component; live vaccines in significant immunosuppression: minor illness is not one.
Q4. A child behind on the schedule: what do you do?	No restarting: continue from where they stopped with a catch-up plan per the Green Book.
Q5. How do you handle firm refusal?	Respect, document, keep the relationship and the door open: the goal is the next conversation, not winning this one.
CURVEBALL	"If vaccines work, why does my vaccinated child need herd immunity?" Answer honestly: no vaccine is 100%: coverage protects the small number in whom protection fails: honesty builds the trust that changes minds.

CHAPTER 54 · PSYCH I: DEPRESSION, ANXIETY & HEALTH ANXIETY

CALM SAFE · RISK ME · MANIA · DEPRESSED · ANXIETY · HEALTH · SIDE EFFECTS · SAFETY · STEP · FIT NOTE

CORE · GREEN PATH · CAUTION — HIGH INSTANT FAIL RISK

Abbreviations used in this chapter: **CBT** Cognitive Behavioural Therapy · **GAD-7** Generalised Anxiety Disorder scale-7 · **MDT** Multidisciplinary Team · **PHQ-9** Patient Health Questionnaire-9 · **SSRI** Selective Serotonin Reuptake Inhibitor

THINK — First Question: "Is this patient safe? Are they at risk of self-harm or suicide?"

Instant Fail Triggers: Not asking about suicide · No safety plan for high-risk · SSRI without bipolar screen · SSRI without side-effect counselling · Reassuring health anxiety excessively

"If you don't ask about suicide, I fail you. Miss bipolar before SSRI = instant fail."

SAY — Golden Minute: "Safety first, then diagnosis, then management. RISK ME → MANIA before SSRI → screen psychosis + physical causes → PHQ-9/GAD-7 → STEP → SIDE EFFECTS counselling → SAFETY plan."

Suicide Risk — RISK ME · Risk Ladder

SAY — Golden Opening: "Before we go further — have you had any thoughts of harming yourself or ending your life?"

R	Recent stressors	"What's been happening recently that's made things worse?"
I	Intent	"Do you actually want to die, or just want the pain to stop?"
S	Specific plan	"Have you thought about how you would do it?"
K	Means	"Do you have access to [method mentioned]?"
M	Motivation (protective factors)	"What keeps you going? What are your reasons to live?"
E	Emergency support	"Who can you call if things get worse?"

Risk	Features	Action
Low	Passive thoughts · no plan	Safety-net + routine follow-up
Moderate	Active thoughts · no plan · some intent	Safety plan + family + 48–72h review
High	Plan + intent + means	Crisis team NOW — do NOT send home alone
Immediate	Actively preparing to die	A&E / 999 — do NOT leave alone

THINK — Screen Before SSRI — MANIA · Psychosis · Physical Causes

MANIA — Screen BEFORE any SSRI (starting SSRI in bipolar can induce mania):
M — Mood elevated/irritable · A — Activity increased · N — Need less sleep · I — Impulsivity (spending/risky) · A — Agrandiosity
If YES to any MANIA question → Do NOT start SSRI without specialist review.

Psychosis Red Flags: Voices when no one around · Paranoia (watching/following) · Delusional guilt → URGENT mental health referral
Physical Causes — rule out before diagnosing: Thyroid · Anaemia · B12/folate · Substance misuse · Medications · Age >65 = organic red flag

DEPRESSED · ANXIETY · PHQ-9/GAD-7

DEPRESSED	ANXIETY
D — Depressed mood	A — Apprehension/worry
E — Energy loss	N — Nervousness
P — Pleasure loss (anhedonia)	X — eXhaustion
R — Retardation/agitation	I — Irritability
E — Eating changes	E — Excessive thoughts (hard to stop)
S — Sleep disturbance	T — Tension (muscle)
S — Self-worth/concentration	Y — sYmptoms (palpitations, sweating)
E — Ending thoughts (SUICIDE)	
D — Duration	

PHQ-9 severity: 5–9 = mild (self-help) · 10–14 = moderate (CBT/consider SSRI) · 15–19 = mod-severe (CBT+SSRI) · 20+ = severe (urgent MH review)
Function: "How are these symptoms affecting your daily life — work, relationships, looking after yourself?" Functional impairment is the key escalation trigger.

Health Anxiety — HEALTH Mnemonic

HEALTH:
H — Health worries persist: "I can see this is really worrying you." · E — Excessive checking (GP visits, internet) · A — AVOID reassurance — validate instead
L — Listen to underlying anxiety · T — Treat with CBT · H — Help patient understand the cycle
Broken Alarm Analogy: "Your body's smoke alarm is too sensitive — if we keep doing tests we just change the batteries. CBT helps retune the alarm."
Avoid: Repeating tests · saying "don't worry" · unqualified reassurance — reinforces the anxiety cycle.

SSRI Counselling — Core 5 · Stepped Care STEP

Core 5 SSRI Side Effects — ALWAYS say all five:
1. Starting (first 1–2 weeks): more anxious/agitated — normal, settles
2. Delayed benefit: 2–4 weeks for full effect — do not stop early
3. Nausea: take with food, usually passes
4. Sexual: can affect sex drive/function — let me know
5. Discontinuation: do not stop suddenly — dizziness, flu-like withdrawal

Also: Continue 6 months after recovery · Under-25 = review in 1 week · Keep medication safe (overdose risk)

Step	Severity	Intervention
1	Mild	Watchful waiting · guided self-help · psychoeducation
2	Mild-moderate	Low-intensity CBT · computerised CBT · group
3	Moderate-severe	High-intensity CBT · counselling · SSRI
4	Severe/complex	Specialist MH · MDT · inpatient if needed

Safety Planning — SAFETY · Sick Note — FIT NOTE

SAFETY — Safety Plan (6 Steps)	FIT NOTE — Sick Note Conversation
S — Spot warning signs: "What thoughts tell you you're heading into crisis?"	F — Function first: "How do your symptoms affect your ability to work?"
A — Ask coping: "What has helped before?"	I — Individualised: "What adjustments might help you return?"
F — Friends/family to call	T — Timeframe: review in [X weeks]
E — Emergency: Samaritans 116 123 · crisis team	N — Not fit vs may be fit with adjustments
T — Take away means: access to medication/weapons	O — Options: phased return · reduced hours · amended duties
Y — Your plan: write together	E — Empathy: "Time off can help, but staying connected to work often aids recovery."

SAY — Language — What to Say · SBAR Escalation

✗ Never Say	✓ Say Instead
"You'll be fine."	"Your symptoms are real and distressing."
"It's just anxiety."	"We'll work on this together."
"Don't worry."	"I can hear how concerned you are."
"Everyone feels like this."	"Many people experience this — you're not alone."
"Nothing is wrong."	"I'm here to support you."

SBAR — Crisis Escalation:
S: "I'm referring a patient with active suicidal ideation and a plan."
B: "[Age] · severe depression · PHQ-9 [score] · lives alone · no social support."
A: "Has thought about [method] · has access · no protective factors."
R: "Need urgent crisis team review — patient cannot go home alone."
Crisis contacts: Samaritans 116 123 (24/7 free) · Crisis team · A&E if immediate risk · 999 if life-threatening

Examiner Checklist

Safety + Assessment ✓	Management ✓
✓ Suicide asked directly	✓ Severity matched to STEP
✓ RISK ME applied	✓ Core 5 SSRI side effects stated
✓ Risk ladder level stated	✓ Bipolar screened BEFORE SSRI
✓ High risk → crisis team, not sent home	✓ Under-25 → 1-week review
✓ Safety plan created if any risk	✓ Health anxiety: no reassurance + CBT
✓ MANIA screen done	✓ Broken alarm analogy used
✓ Psychosis screened	✓ FIT NOTE options discussed
✓ Physical causes ruled out	✓ SAFETY plan documented
✓ PHQ-9/GAD-7 referenced	✓ Samaritans 116 123 given
✓ Function explored	✓ Follow-up arranged + safety-net

Final Exam Mantra

Safety first → RISK ME → Risk ladder: Low=outpatient · Moderate=48-72h · High=crisis NOW · Immediate=999
MANIA before SSRI · Psychosis screen · Physical causes (thyroid/anaemia/B12/substances)
PHQ-9/GAD-7 + DEPRESSED/ANXIETY · Function is the key escalation trigger
Core 5 SSRI: activation · delay · nausea · sexual · discontinuation · STEP 1–4
Health anxiety: validate · no reassurance · broken alarm · CBT · FIT NOTE: options + adjustments

Gold Closing:
"Risk assessed using RISK ME — [low/moderate/high]. MANIA screened. Psychosis and physical causes excluded. PHQ-9 score [X] — Step [X] care. [If SSRI:] Counselled on core 5 side effects. [If health anxiety:] Validated, avoiding reassurance, CBT signposted. Safety plan created. Review in [X weeks]. Samaritans 116 123 given. If feels unsafe — A&E or 999."

Ask suicide directly first question always	RISK ME 6-step risk assessment	High risk = crisis NOW not sent home alone	MANIA before SSRI miss = instant fail	Core 5 SSRI always counsel all 5
No reassurance HA broken alarm + CBT	PHQ-9 / GAD-7 severity thresholds	STEP 1-4 match severity to care	Samaritans 116 123 24/7 safety net	FIT NOTE options adjustments not dismissal

TOP 5 EXAMINER Q&A · PSYCH I · DEPRESSION & ANXIETY	
Q1. Core questions in any depression assessment?	Low mood, anhedonia and fatigue over two weeks, biological symptoms, functional impact: and always a direct risk assessment.
Q2. How do you ask about suicide?	Directly and without euphemism: "Have you had thoughts of ending your life?": asking does not plant the idea.
Q3. What is stepped care?	Matching intervention intensity to severity: from active monitoring and guided self-help through talking therapies to medication and specialist care.
Q4. Starting an SSRI: what must you counsel?	Two to four weeks to effect, early side effects, possible initial anxiety, not addictive, do not stop suddenly: review within 1–2 weeks (1 week if under 30).
Q5. Health anxiety: what maintains it and what helps?	Repeated reassurance and checking maintain the cycle: explanation plus CBT breaks it: more tests are not treatment.
CURVEBALL	"I would never do anything, I have kids" said while avoiding eye contact. Protective factors are noted, not banked: explore passive ideation, plans and means anyway: gentle persistence over polite acceptance.

CHAPTER 55 · PSYCH II: ALCOHOL MISUSE, SELF-HARM & SUICIDAL RISK

ASSESS · SAD PERSONS · 4 Suicide Drivers · Hopelessness Ladder · Intent Matrix · Safety Triangle

CORE · GREEN PATH · CAUTION — CRITICAL INSTANT FAIL RISK

Abbreviations used in this chapter: **MHA** Mental Health Act

THINK — First Question: "Is this patient at immediate risk? Do they need urgent medical treatment? Do I need psychiatry NOW?"

Core Rules: Medical stability FIRST · Behaviour overrides verbal denial · Calm/smiling after attempt = HIGHEST RISK · Hopelessness > intent · Uncertainty = ADMIT

Instant Fail Triggers: Miss Wernicke's · Glucose before thiamine (if Wernicke's risk) · Discharge self-harm without psychosocial assessment · SAD PERSONS to rule out suicide · No safety plan · Leaving patient alone

SAY — Golden Minute: "Medical first → ASSESS framework → 3 core questions → hopelessness ladder → 4 drivers → planning spectrum → intent matrix → risk formulation → safety plan → discharge triangle."

1. Alcohol Misuse · Wernicke's · Delirium Tremens

Wernicke's Encephalopathy — DO NOT MISS:

Classic triad: Confusion + Ataxia + Nystagmus — ALL THREE NOT ALWAYS PRESENT

3 questions (any YES = give thiamine): Malnourished? · Vomiting? · Heavy drinking for years?

IV Pabrinex immediately — do NOT wait for confirmation. Thiamine BEFORE glucose (unless hypoglycaemic — then treat hypoglycaemia first then thiamine immediately).

Prophylaxis: Oral thiamine 100mg TDS in all high-risk patients (chronic alcohol, malnutrition, vomiting)

4 Cs of Alcohol Dependence: Compulsion · Control (lost) · Cutting down (failed) · Continued use despite harm

Withdrawal Red Flags: Previous seizures · Previous DTs · High daily intake · Concurrent benzodiazepines → monitor closely

Delirium Tremens: Confusion + severe agitation + hallucinations (visual/tactile) + autonomic instability → HDU/ICU consideration

2. Suicidal Risk — 3 Core Questions · 4 Drivers · Hopelessness Ladder

3 Core Questions — Anchor Every Assessment:

1. "Did you want to die at the time?" → suicidal intent
2. "Did you plan it?" → severity + organisation
3. "Do you still feel unsafe now?" → ongoing risk — can change rapidly

4 Suicide Drivers:
Burden ("people are better off without me") · Belongingness failure (isolation/rejection) · Capability (fearlessness/past attempts) · Hopelessness = STRONGEST predictor
Alcohol multiplier: Alcohol increases suicide risk 7-fold · Alcohol + depression = 37-fold

Level	Hopelessness Statement	Risk
0	"I know things will improve."	Low
1	"I'm not sure things will improve."	Moderate
2	"I can't see things improving."	High
3	"Nothing will ever change."	Very high
4	"There is no point in living."	EMERGENCY

Planning Spectrum: Vague → semi-structured → structured (saved tablets) → OPERATIONAL (time/place chosen) = EMERGENCY
Intent Matrix: Desire to die × belief attempt would kill. High × High = VERY HIGH RISK
Behavioural Rule: Behaviour contradicts verbal reassurance → prioritise behaviour. Denial ≠ safety.
Quiet Patient Rule: Calm · quiet · resigned · or suddenly smiling after attempt = HIGHEST RISK. Do NOT be falsely reassured.

Suicide Scripts — Coded Language (probe immediately):
"I'm done." · "I won't be here much longer." · "Everyone will be better off." · "I've sorted everything out." · "What's the point?"

3. Psychosocial Assessment · Risk Formulation · SAD PERSONS

Domain	Key Questions
Episode details	What happened? What taken/done? When? Where?
Intent + lethality	Wanted to die? How lethal? Avoided discovery? Prepared?
Self-harm function	To die · cope · punish · communicate · dissociation?
Protective factors	What kept you from more serious harm? What do you look forward to?
Ongoing thoughts	Do you still feel like hurting yourself NOW?
Support	Who is at home? Who can supervise tonight?
Risk escalators	Recent discharge · anniversary · bereavement · financial/legal · housing loss

SAD PERSONS: Memory prompt ONLY. LOW SENSITIVITY — nearly half of suicides score low. Clinical judgement predominates.
4P Risk Formulation: Predisposing (background) · Precipitating (triggers) · Perpetuating (maintaining) · Protective (strengths)
Stress-test protective factors: "How confident this keeps you safe? What if support isn't available? What if you feel worse tonight?"

4. Capacity · Safety Plan · Discharge Safety Triangle

Capacity — MCA 4 Principles: Understand · Retain · Weigh · Communicate — decision-specific AND time-specific
Pitfalls: Intoxicated = cannot assess reliably · Depression impairs weighing · Delirium = no capacity · Personality disorder ≠ lack of capacity
MHA: Risk to self or others + mental disorder + needs hospital treatment + no less restrictive option. Least restrictive first — but do NOT delay if safety demands.

Step	Safety Plan Element	3 Means Restriction Questions
1	Recognise warning signs	"Who will remove medications/sharps at home?"
2	Internal coping (things they can do alone)	"Is there someone who can stay with you tonight?"
3	Social contacts who can distract	"Do you have access to weapons, ligatures, or high places?"
4	Family/friends who can help in crisis	
5	Crisis: team · GP · 111 · 999	
6	Means restriction: lock meds · remove sharps/belts/shoelaces	

Discharge Safety Triangle — ALL 3 must be present before discharge:
1. Internal safety (no current intent) · 2. External safety (supervision + means restriction) · 3. Professional safety (follow-up arranged)
Reassess risk immediately BEFORE discharge — intent can change within minutes.
Safety net failure: Support overwhelmed/absent/intoxicated · patient lives alone · no follow-up · patient minimises despite evidence · no phone/transport

Follow-up by risk: High = admit · Moderate = crisis team + 24–48h review · Lower = GP within 1 week + crisis numbers

Examiner Checklist

Alcohol + Assessment ✓	Risk + Disposition ✓
✓ 3 Wernicke's questions + IV Pabrinex if yes	✓ 3 core questions asked
✓ Thiamine before glucose (unless hypo)	✓ Hopelessness ladder used

Alcohol + Assessment ✓	Risk + Disposition ✓
✓ Withdrawal red flags assessed	✓ 4 suicide drivers assessed
✓ DTs recognised + escalated	✓ Planning spectrum assessed
✓ Medical stability confirmed first	✓ Behaviour rule applied
✓ Glucose checked in all confused/SH	✓ Quiet/smiling patient rule stated
✓ MCA capacity assessed	✓ SAD PERSONS as prompt only
✓ MHA considered	✓ Safety plan: collaborative + means restriction
✓ Confidentiality explained	✓ Discharge triangle: all 3 confirmed
✓ Risk reassessed before discharge	✓ Uncertainty = ADMIT stated

Final Exam Mantra

Medical FIRST · Glucose in ALL · Wernicke's = Pabrinex NOW · Thiamine before glucose (unless hypo)

3 core questions · 4 suicide drivers · Hopelessness > intent · Behaviour overrides denial · Calm/smiling = highest risk

Planning spectrum: operational = EMERGENCY · Alcohol multiplier: 7-fold (37-fold with depression)

SAD PERSONS = prompt only · Stress-test protective factors · Discharge triangle: internal + external + professional

Reassess before discharge · Uncertainty = ADMIT

Gold Closing:

"Medical stability confirmed. ASSESS framework applied. 3 core questions: intent, planning, current safety. Hopelessness level [X]. 4 drivers assessed. Planning spectrum: [level]. Behaviour rule: [consistent/contradicts]. Risk formulated: 4P model. Capacity: [intact/impaired]. Safety plan collaborative with means restriction. Discharge triangle: [met/not met]. Reassessed before discharge. Uncertainty = admitting."

Medical FIRST before psychiatric assess	Wernicke's = Pabrinex IV now, do not wait	Thiamine before glucose unless hypoglycaemic	3 core questions intent, plan, current safe	Hopelessness > intent strongest predictor
Behaviour overrides denial ≠ safety	Calm/smiling = risk do not be reassured	SAD PERSONS prompt only, not rule-out	Discharge triangle all 3 must be present	Uncertainty = ADMIT always

TOP 5 EXAMINER Q&A · PSYCH II · ALCOHOL, SELF-HARM & SUICIDAL RISK

Q1. What does SAD PERSONS-style risk assessment actually require?	A structured conversation: ideation, plan, means, intent, protective factors and mental state: scores never replace judgement.

TOP 5 EXAMINER Q&A · PSYCH II · ALCOHOL, SELF-HARM & SUICIDAL RISK	
Q2. After self-harm, what must happen before discharge?	Psychosocial assessment, capacity check, safety planning, means restriction discussion and follow-up arrangement: never discharge unassessed.
Q3. What is in a safety plan?	Warning signs, personal coping strategies, contacts for support, professional and crisis numbers, and an agreed plan for access to means.
Q4. Alcohol withdrawal: who needs inpatient detox?	History of seizures or delirium tremens, severe dependence, comorbidity or failed community detox: give thiamine either way.
Q5. What is delirium tremens and its treatment?	Agitation, confusion, hallucinations and autonomic storm 48–72 hours after stopping: benzodiazepines per protocol, it is life-threatening.
CURVEBALL	He is intoxicated now and says he wants to die. Intoxication invalidates neither risk nor your duty: keep him safe, reassess when sober, and never discharge a suicidal intoxicated patient into the night.

CHAPTER 56 · PSYCH III: DNACPR, PALLIATIVE CARE & END-OF-LIFE PLANNING

DNACPR · CPR REALITY · LEGAL · LPA-AD · URWC · PAIN · SYRINGE · SPIKES · CEILING · AMBER

CORE · CAUTION — INSTANT FAIL RISK · HIGH STAKES

Abbreviations used in this chapter: **ACS** Acute Coronary Syndrome · **ADRT** Advance Decision to Refuse Treatment · **AKI** Acute Kidney Injury · **AVPU** Alert, Voice, Pain, Unresponsive · **BNF** British National Formulary · **CAP** Community-Acquired Pneumonia · **CKD** Chronic Kidney Disease · **COPD** Chronic Obstructive Pulmonary Disease · **CPM** Central Pontine Myelinolysis · **CRT** Capillary Refill Time · **DKA** Diabetic Ketoacidosis · **DNACPR** Do Not Attempt Cardiopulmonary Resuscitation · **DVLA** Driver & Vehicle Licensing Agency · **FRIII** Fixed Rate Intravenous Insulin Infusion · **GTN** Glyceryl Trinitrate · **HAP** Hospital-Acquired Pneumonia · **HGV** Heavy Goods Vehicle · **HHS** Hyperosmolar Hyperglycaemic State · **ICD** Implantable Cardioverter Defibrillator · **LP** Lumbar Puncture · **LPA** Lasting Power of Attorney · **MDT** Multidisciplinary Team · **MRSA** Meticillin-Resistant Staphylococcus aureus · **MTX** Methotrexate · **NEWS2** National Early Warning Score 2 · **NIV** Non-Invasive Ventilation · **PCC** Prothrombin Complex Concentrate · **PCI** Percutaneous Coronary Intervention · **PE** Pulmonary Embolism · **PEA** Pulseless Electrical Activity · **PID** Pelvic Inflammatory Disease · **PLAB** Professional & Linguistic Assessments Board · **PPI** Proton Pump Inhibitor · **ROSC** Return of Spontaneous Circulation · **RSI** Rapid Sequence Induction · **SBP** Systolic Blood Pressure · **STEMI** ST-Elevation Myocardial Infarction · **TCA** Tricyclic Antidepressant · **URTI** Upper Respiratory Tract Infection · **VF** Ventricular Fibrillation · **VRIII** Variable Rate Intravenous Insulin Infusion

DISTINCTION — Golden Triad of Fail:

1. Saying "Do Not Resuscitate" without explaining CPR reality
2. Confusing Lasting Power of Attorney with Advance Decision
3. Ignoring family distress or leaving no space for questions

Instant Fail Triggers: Say DNR without CPR reality · Present as "stopping treatment" · Confuse LPA with AD · Can't name 5 drugs · No syringe driver knowledge · No documentation reasoning

SAY — Golden Minute: "DNACPR = CPR-only. All other care continues. LPA = Lets Person Act. AD = Already Decided. We're not stopping care — we're changing focus to comfort and dignity."

SAY — 1. The DNACPR Conversation · CPR Reality · What Continues

D	Discuss goals first	"What matters most to you?"
N	Never say "DNR" alone	Always explain CPR reality first
A	Assess capacity using URWC	Before any discussion
C	CPR reality	Broken ribs · ICU · rarely successful
P	Patient/family views	"What do you understand? What matters?"
R	Review + document	Reasoning · who consulted · review date

CPR REALITY — Say All of This:
"CPR involves pushing very hard on the chest — can break ribs. Not like on TV. If it works, they'd need intensive care on a breathing machine. In frailty/advanced illness it is very unlikely to work and often causes harm. Even when CPR works, people rarely return to their previous independence. Survivors often have brain injury and a prolonged ICU stay."

✓ CONTINUES after DNACPR	✗ DOES NOT CONTINUE
Oxygen	CPR — that is ALL that stops
Antibiotics	Nothing else is affected
IV/SC fluids (if appropriate)	
All pain relief and comfort measures	
All nursing care	
Treatment of reversible causes	

ReSPECT form: Patient values · clinical recommendations · CPR decision · escalation limits (ICU, NIV, ward)
Futile CPR: Consultant can make DNACPR decision even if family disagree — must document clearly and offer second opinion
When NOT to discuss: Would cause significant psychological harm · patient actively dying/unconscious · patient refuses — document and revisit

2. Legal Framework — LEGAL · LPA vs Advance Decision · URWC · CEILING

LPA vs Advance Decision — MUST NOT CONFUSE:
LPA = Lets Person Act: Appoints someone to decide when patient lacks capacity. Must be registered for health/welfare.
AD = Already Decided: Refuses specific treatments in advance. Written when patient had capacity. Life-sustaining: must be written, signed, witnessed, explicit. Legally binding if valid and applicable.
ADRT validity check: Valid (not withdrawn)? · Applicable (current situation matches)? · Specific? · Signed + witnessed?

URWC — Capacity Assessment (any one failed = lacks capacity):
U — Understand · R — Retain · W — Weigh · C — Communicate
Assume capacity unless evidence otherwise. Fluctuating capacity: involve patient at capable times.

CEILING — Treatment Escalation (discuss beyond CPR):
C — CPR · E — Escalation (ICU/HDU) · I — Infections (antibiotics) · L — Liquids (IV/SC fluids) · I — Interventions (NIV/O_2) · N — Nutrition · G — Goals of care (reviewed daily)

AMBER Care Bundle (deteriorating patients): Assess · Meet (MDT) · Be clear (honest) · Escalate (plan) · Review (daily)

Documentation must include: Patient details · clinical reasoning · who consulted · capacity status · review date · senior signature · communicated to GP

3. Palliative Care · 5 Drugs · Syringe Driver

Symptom	First-Line Drug	Notes
Pain	Morphine	Start low · titrate · breakthrough PRN (1/6 total daily dose)
Breathlessness	Low-dose morphine	Add midazolam if anxiety prominent
Agitation/restlessness	Midazolam	PRN · levomepromazine if refractory
Nausea/vomiting	Haloperidol	Levomepromazine if first-line fails
Secretions	Glycopyrronium	Or hyoscine butylbromide

PAIN Opioid Principles:
P — Percentage: breakthrough = 1/6 of total daily dose · A — Antiemetic: always co-prescribe · I — Increase if uncontrolled · N — Needs syringe driver if unable to swallow
"I will prescribe anticipatory subcutaneous medications for all 5 symptoms so nurses can give them urgently."

SYRINGE Driver Script:
"A small battery-powered pump giving medication continuously through a tiny needle under the skin. No repeated injections. Drugs run steadily. We combine drugs for pain, agitation, or secretions. Nurse checks regularly and we adjust. Very common in the last days of life when people can't swallow. Won't hurt — just for comfort."
Syringe driver = steady background control. For acute distress — give PRN doses first.
Not euthanasia: "A syringe driver does not hasten death — it gives comfort and prevents suffering."

4. Family Communication — SPIKES · Difficult Moments · Misconceptions

S	Setting	Private room · sit down · tissues · no interruptions
P	Perception	"What's your understanding of what's happening?"
I	Invitation	"Would it be OK if I share my thoughts?"
K	Knowledge	Clear · honest · no jargon
E	Emotions	"I can see this is very difficult." — validate — leave silence
S	Strategy/Summary	Summarise plan · check understanding · next steps

Difficult Moments — Scripts:
"So you're letting them die?" → "We're not causing their death. The illness is. Our role is to prevent suffering and respect their dignity."
"How long?" → "I can't say exactly — it could be days, but we'll keep them comfortable throughout."
Anger → "I can hear how upset you are. This is incredibly difficult." Silence — stay silent, wait, don't fill the space.
Fluids/feeding → "In the last days, the body can't absorb fluids well. Forced fluids can cause discomfort. We focus on mouth care and comfort."

Misconception	What It Actually Means
DNACPR = stopping treatment	DNACPR = one thing only: no CPR. ALL other care continues.
DNACPR = no ICU or NIV	ICU and NIV are SEPARATE decisions — documented separately
DNACPR = giving up	Focusing care on what will actually help
Syringe driver = hastening death	Gives comfort — does not hasten death
Palliative care = end of life only	Can run alongside disease-modifying treatment

Examiner Checklist

DNACPR + Legal ✓	Drugs + Communication ✓
✓ CPR reality: ribs + ICU + rarely works	✓ Pain: morphine named
✓ DNACPR = CPR-only stated	✓ Breathlessness: low-dose morphine
✓ All other care continues stated	✓ Agitation: midazolam named
✓ CEILING discussed (not just CPR)	✓ Nausea: haloperidol named
✓ ReSPECT form mentioned	✓ Secretions: glycopyrronium named
✓ URWC capacity assessed	✓ Antiemetic co-prescribed with opioids
✓ LPA vs AD distinction clear	✓ Anticipatory prescribing mentioned
✓ ADRT validity check stated	✓ Syringe driver explained (SYRINGE)
✓ Documentation: reasoning + review date	✓ SPIKES applied + silence used
✓ Senior involvement if conflict	✓ Misconceptions addressed proactively

Final Exam Mantra

DNACPR = CPR-only · all other care continues · CPR REALITY: ribs + ICU + rarely works
LPA = Lets Person Act · AD = Already Decided · ADRT: valid + applicable + specific + signed
URWC: Understand, Retain, Weigh, Communicate · CEILING: not just CPR · AMBER: deteriorating
5 drugs: morphine · morphine · midazolam · haloperidol · glycopyrronium
SYRINGE driver = comfort not death · SPIKES + silence is gold · 7 misconceptions

Gold Closing:
"DNACPR = CPR-only, all other care continues. CPR reality given. CEILING discussed. URWC capacity assessed. LPA vs AD distinction made, ADRT validity checked. 5 drugs prescribed anticipatorily. Syringe driver explained. SPIKES applied, silence used, distress acknowledged. Documentation: reasoning, who consulted, review date, senior signature."

DNACPR = CPR only all other care continues	CPR reality ribs + ICU + rarely works	LPA = Lets Person Act AD = Already Decided	ADRT validity valid, applicable, specific	URWC capacity all 4 to have capacity
CEILING beyond CPR planning	5 drugs morphine morphine midaz halop glyco	Antiemetic always with every opioid	Syringe driver comfort not hastening death	Silence is gold SPIKES + wait

TOP 5 EXAMINER Q&A · PSYCH III · DNACPR, PALLIATIVE & END-OF-LIFE	
Q1. What is a DNACPR decision legally?	A clinical decision about a treatment (CPR), made with consultation, not consent: but failing to discuss it is unlawful absent good reason.
Q2. Who decides when the patient lacks capacity?	The senior clinician, in best interests, consulting family and any LPA for health and welfare: an LPA with authority can refuse treatment.
Q3. What goes through a syringe driver at end of life?	Continuous subcutaneous symptom control: typically an opioid, antiemetic, anxiolytic and antisecretory as needed.
Q4. How does SPIKES structure bad news?	Setting, Perception, Invitation, Knowledge, Empathy, Strategy/Summary: warn before the news and chunk information.
Q5. What do you say about stopping treatment?	We never stop caring: the goal changes from cure to comfort: nutrition, dignity and symptom control continue.
CURVEBALL	The family demands "do everything" for a dying patient with a valid DNACPR. Hear the love inside the demand, explain CPR's reality in this body, and hold the clinical line with compassion: comfort is doing everything.

Appendix 2A

PLAB 2 ACUTE ALGORITHM QUICK REFERENCE

A–E First · Escalate Early · Reassess After Every Intervention · Treat Life Threats Before Diagnosis

High-yield acute algorithms · Word-for-word examiner language · First-action table · Emergency safety triggers

KEY — Universal First Step — Say This First in Every Emergency

"I would assess the patient using an A–E approach, call for senior help early, attach monitoring, give oxygen if hypoxic (target SpO_2 94–98%, or 88–92% if COPD risk), and gain IV access."

ABCDE Universal Framework

Step	Assessment	Immediate Actions	Always Verbalise
A	Airway: Patent? Obstructed?	Head-tilt chin-lift · Jaw thrust · Suction · Adjuncts	Airway status
B	Breathing: RR · SpO_2 · Chest movement	O_2 if hypoxic (94–98% / 88–92% COPD) · Inspect · Percuss · Auscultate	Oxygen target
C	Circulation: HR · BP · Perfusion	2 large-bore IVs · Bloods · Fluids if indicated	IV access + bloods
D	Disability: GCS/AVPU · Glucose · Pupils	Check glucose · Neuro assessment · Temperature	Glucose result
E	Exposure: Full examination	Top-to-toe while preserving dignity	Senior escalation

Exam Performance Rules:
Say A–E first — shows structure · Escalate early — demonstrates safe practice
Treat life threats before diagnosis — prevents dangerous delays · Reassess after every intervention — closed-loop safety
Speak calmly and clearly — leadership under pressure

PLAB 2 First-Action Table

Condition	First Action
Sepsis	Sepsis Six within 1 hour
Anaphylaxis	IM adrenaline 0.5 mg (1:1000) into anterolateral thigh

Condition	First Action
Cardiac arrest	Start CPR 30:2 immediately
Status epilepticus	IV lorazepam 4 mg (or buccal midazolam if no IV)
ACS	ECG + Aspirin 300 mg chewed
Stroke	FAST + urgent non-contrast CT head
DKA	IV 0.9% saline 1 L in first hour
Acute severe asthma	Oxygen + salbutamol nebuliser (O_2-driven)
Testicular torsion	Call urology immediately — do NOT wait for ultrasound
Fournier's gangrene	Urgent surgical referral + IV antibiotics
Paraphimosis	Immediate reduction (ice · compression · sugar gauze)
Acute urinary retention	Exclude urethral injury, then catheterise (5 Cs)
Hyperkalaemia	IV calcium gluconate (if ECG changes)
Hypoglycaemia	IV 10% glucose (or oral if conscious)
Upper GI bleed	2 large-bore IV cannulas + crossmatch
TCA overdose	A–E + continuous ECG monitoring

Sepsis — Sepsis Six (Within 1 Hour)

#	Action
1	Blood cultures BEFORE antibiotics
2	IV broad-spectrum antibiotics
3	IV fluids
4	Lactate
5	Urine output monitoring
6	Oxygen if hypoxic

> "Source control is essential — relieve obstruction, drain abscess, or remove infected lines. Antibiotics alone are NOT sufficient."
> "I will reassess after every intervention – if no improvement, escalate to ICU."
> "I would not delay antibiotics beyond one hour."

Anaphylaxis — Resuscitation Council UK

Sudden airway/breathing/circulation compromise ± rash → adrenaline first.

✓ IM adrenaline 0.5 mg (0.5 mL of 1:1000) into anterolateral thigh — IMMEDIATELY

✓ Repeat every 5 min if needed · ✓ Lay flat + legs elevated · ✓ High-flow O_2

✓ IV fluids · ✓ Chlorphenamine + hydrocortisone AFTER adrenaline · ✓ Observe 6–12 hours for biphasic

"I would never delay adrenaline."

Cardiac Arrest — Adult ALS

Rhythm	Action
Shockable (VF/pVT)	Shock → CPR 2 min → Adrenaline 1 mg IV after 3rd shock
Non-shockable (PEA/Asystole)	CPR → Adrenaline 1 mg IV immediately

4 Hs	4 Ts
Hypoxia	Tension pneumothorax
Hypovolaemia	Cardiac tamponade
Hypo/hyperkalaemia + metabolic	Toxins
Hypothermia	Thrombosis (PE/coronary)

After ROSC: Optimise oxygenation · BP support · ICU · "I would treat reversible causes and reassess continuously."

Status Epilepticus

Step	Action
1	A–E + oxygen + left lateral position
2	Check glucose immediately
3	IV lorazepam 4 mg
4	Repeat once after 10 minutes if ongoing
5	Second-line: levetiracetam or phenytoin
6	Refractory seizures → RSI + ICU

If no IV access: Buccal midazolam 10 mg
"I would protect the airway and note time zero. I will reassess after every intervention."

ACS · Stroke — Core Actions

Condition	Immediate Actions	Must-Say
ACS	A–E + monitoring · ECG immediately · Aspirin 300 mg chewed · GTN if SBP >90 · Consider ticagrelor + anticoagulation	"Escalate urgently to cardiology."
Stroke	FAST + A–E · Check glucose · Urgent CT head · Thrombolysis if ≤4.5 h · Swallow screen · Stroke team	"Time is brain — I would not delay imaging."

DKA · Acute Severe Asthma

DKA: A–E + senior · IV 0.9% saline 1L/hr · FRIII 0.1 units/kg/hr · Glucose <14 → add 10% dextrose · Identify precipitant · "Never stop insulin early."

Asthma: O_2 + salbutamol neb (O_2-driven) · Add ipratropium · Prednisolone 40–50 mg PO or IV hydrocortisone · IV magnesium if life-threatening · Early ICU · "Never sedate an asthmatic."

Never Miss in Asthma: Silent chest · Rising CO_2 · Exhaustion

High-Yield Surgical Emergencies

Testicular Torsion: "Time is testis — 6-hour window." Call urology within 2 min. Do NOT wait for US. Manual detorsion (outward rotation). Previous orchidopexy does NOT exclude torsion.

Fournier's Gangrene: Surgical referral + IV antibiotics + fluids + glucose check. Examine FULL perineum, perianal, buttocks, inner thighs.

Paraphimosis: Ice → compression → sugar gauze → manual reduction → Dundee technique → urology dorsal slit.

Urinary Retention: Exclude urethral injury first. 5 Cs. Monitor post-obstructive diuresis (>200 mL/hr for 2h → inform urology — life-threatening hypovolaemia risk).

Metabolic Emergencies

Condition	Step 1	Steps 2–3
Hyperkalaemia	IV calcium gluconate (cardiac stabilisation)	Insulin+glucose · Salbutamol → Furosemide · Dialysis if severe
Hypoglycaemia	<4 mmol/L + symptoms	Conscious → oral glucose 15–20g · Unconscious → IV 10% glucose OR IM glucagon. Recheck in 10 min.

Upper GI Bleed · TCA Overdose

Upper GI Bleed: A–E · 2 large-bore IVs · FBC+U&E+Coagulation+Crossmatch · Restrictive transfusion (1 unit, reassess) · Reverse anticoagulation · IV PPI · Variceal: terlipressin + IV ceftriaxone + urgent endoscopy

TCA Overdose: A–E · Continuous ECG monitoring · IV sodium bicarbonate if QRS >100–120 ms or arrhythmia · "NEVER give flumazenil."

Never / Always Rules

Condition	✗ Never
Anaphylaxis	Never delay adrenaline
DKA	Never stop insulin early
Asthma	Never sedate
TCA overdose	Never give flumazenil
Testicular torsion	Never delay urology for ultrasound
Urethral injury	Never catheterise if blood at meatus or pelvic fracture

KEY — High-Yield Examiner Lines

Context	Phrase
Sepsis	"I would not delay antibiotics beyond one hour."
Sepsis — source control	"Source control is essential — antibiotics alone are not sufficient."
Sepsis — reassess	"I will reassess after every intervention — if no improvement, escalate to ICU."
Seizure	"I would protect the airway and note time zero."
Cardiac arrest	"I would treat reversible causes."
Torsion	"Time is testis — previous orchidopexy does NOT exclude torsion."
Fournier's	"Urgent surgical debridement required — examine full perineum."
Urinary retention	"I will monitor for post-obstructive diuresis."

Final Takeaway — What the Examiner Looks For

Examiner Looks For	Your Response
Structure	A–E first
Safety	Oxygen + IV access + monitoring
Leadership	Escalate early
Prioritisation	Treat life threats first
Closed-loop care	Reassess after every intervention
Professionalism	Calm, clear delegation

Final Instructions:

- Memorise the Universal First Step cold.
- Memorise the First-Action Table cold.
- Always verbalise escalation and reassessment.
- Treat life threats before diagnosis.
- Never break the Never/Always rules.

A–E first every emergency, every time	Universal line say it cold	Escalate early before full diagnosis	Reassess always after every intervention	Adrenaline never delay in anaphylaxis
Sepsis Six within 1 hour	Source control antibiotics alone not enough	Time is testis no imaging delay in torsion	Never sedate asthma absolute rule	Never flumazenil TCA overdose rule

Appendix 2B · DVLA FITNESS TO DRIVE — QUICK REFERENCE

Neurological · Cardiovascular · Syncope · Diabetes · Visual · Sleep · Alcohol · Medications

Group 1 (cars & motorcycles) · Group 2 (HGV/bus) rules are ALWAYS stricter

DISTINCTION — Golden Rule: "If a medical condition may affect safe driving, the patient must stop driving immediately."
Patient's legal responsibility to notify DVLA. Your role: advise clearly and DOCUMENT in the medical record.

OSCE Gold Script: "For safety reasons you should avoid driving for the recommended period. It is your legal responsibility to inform the DVLA, and I will document that we discussed this today."
S-H-D-V-S (High-Risk Five): S=Seizure · H=Hypoglycaemia risk · D=Dangerous arrhythmia · V=Visual field defect · S=Sleep apnoea (severe) → consider DVLA notification

Neurological Conditions

Condition	Stop Driving	Notify DVLA?	Key Points
First unprovoked seizure	6 months	✓ YES	Established epilepsy requires 12 months seizure-free; a first single seizure requires 6 months (12 if investigations show increased risk).
Epilepsy / recurrent seizures	12 months seizure-free	✓ YES	Must meet seizure-free requirement
Single TIA	1 month	✗ NO	Notify only if deficit persists at 1 month
Established stroke	1 month	✗ NO	Notify if neurological deficit remains
Stroke-related seizure	6–12 months	✓ YES	Depends if provoked/unprovoked
Crescendo or recurrent TIA	Until specialist review	✓ YES	Higher stroke risk

Cardiovascular Conditions

Condition	Stop Driving	Notify DVLA?	Key Points
MI treated with PCI / stent	1 week	✗ NO	If recovery uncomplicated
MI without PCI or complicated MI	4 weeks	✗ NO	Longer if complications
Elective PCI / stent	1 week	✗ NO	Must be symptom-free

Condition	Stop Driving	Notify DVLA?	Key Points
CABG surgery	4 weeks	✗ NO	Must be clinically stable
Pacemaker insertion	1 week	✓ YES	Patient must inform DVLA
ICD — primary prevention	1 month	✓ YES	Implanted before any arrhythmic event
ICD — secondary prevention	6 months	✓ YES	After VT/VF or aborted cardiac arrest
Arrhythmia causing syncope	Until controlled	✓ YES	Includes AF with syncope risk
Angina	While symptomatic	✗ NO	Must stop if symptoms at rest or while driving

Syncope · Diabetes

Syncope	Stop Driving	Notify DVLA?
Syncope — cause identified and treated	4 weeks	✗ NO
Syncope — no cause identified	6 months	✓ YES

Diabetes	Notify DVLA?	Key Points
Insulin-treated diabetes	✓ YES	Must monitor glucose before driving
Impaired hypoglycaemia awareness	✓ YES	Must not drive until awareness restored
Severe hypoglycaemia requiring assistance	✓ YES	Must inform DVLA
Non-insulin diabetes (diet/tablets)	✗ NO	Notify only if complications affect driving

Visual · Sleep · Alcohol · Sedating Medications

Visual: Number plate at 20m (with aids if needed). Any visual field defect affecting safe driving → notify DVLA.

Sleep apnoea: Obstructive sleep apnoea with excessive daytime sleepiness → notify DVLA + avoid driving until controlled.

Alcohol/drugs: Alcohol dependence → notify DVLA. Drug misuse affecting driving → notify DVLA.

Sedating medications: Must not drive if sedated. Warn at prescribing + document. Opioids · benzodiazepines · antihistamines · antipsychotics (initiation). Check BNF if in doubt.

Hypoglycaemia While Driving — Immediate Actions

1. Stop the vehicle as soon as it is safe.
2. Remove keys from ignition.
3. Move to passenger seat.
4. Take fast-acting carbohydrates.
5. Do NOT drive again until glucose is normal AND symptoms resolved.

Exam tip: "Keys from ignition" and "passenger seat" commonly missed. Both criteria required: glucose normal AND symptoms resolved.

Must-Notify Shortlist · Exam-Morning Reference

Must Notify DVLA	Exam-Morning: Stop Duration
Seizure / epilepsy (any seizure)	First seizure: 6 months stop ✓ notify
Stroke / TIA: deficit persisting >1 month	TIA: 1 month stop ✗ (unless deficit persists)
Insulin-treated diabetes (ongoing)	Stroke: 1 month stop ✗ (unless deficit persists)
Severe hypoglycaemia requiring assistance	MI + PCI/stent: 1 week stop ✗ notify
Visual field loss affecting driving	MI no stent: 4 weeks stop ✗ notify
Dangerous arrhythmia with syncope/incapacity	Insulin diabetes: no stop period ✓ notify
Severe sleep apnoea with daytime sleepiness	ICD: 1 month primary · 6 months secondary ✓ notify
Alcohol dependence / drug misuse	Pacemaker: 1 week stop ✓ notify

Key Pattern: Notify DVLA = Seizure · ICD · Pacemaker · Insulin · Arrhythmia with syncope · Visual field · Sleep apnoea

Post-procedure: General anaesthetic or sedation = avoid driving for 48 hours. Minor procedures without sedation = safe once fully recovered.

Final Takeaway

Advise stop driving · State correct duration · Explain legal duty to notify DVLA · Document the advice

Group 2 (HGV/bus) rules are ALWAYS stricter — flag this whenever relevant

S-H-D-V-S: Seizure · Hypoglycaemia · Dangerous arrhythmia · Visual field defect · Sleep apnoea

Script: "Stop driving now. Legal duty to notify DVLA. I will document this conversation today."

First seizure 6 months + notify DVLA	TIA / stroke 1 month (no notify unless deficit)	MI + PCI 1 week (no notify)	ICD 1 month primary · 6 months secondary	Insulin diabetes notify DVLA always
Hypo while driving keys out + passenger seat	Visual field loss notify DVLA always	Sleep apnoea severe notify DVLA always	Sedating meds warn + document always	GA / sedation 48 hours no driving

Appendix 2C · ANTIBIOTIC PRESCRIBING ESSENTIALS

BNF/NICE aligned · OSCE-optimised · Sepsis Protocol · Stewardship · Allergy Alternatives

CORE · HIGH STAKES · Acute · Prescribing Stations

Instant Fail: Prescribing without allergy check · Wrong antibiotic for infection site · Delaying antibiotics in sepsis · Missing stewardship review · Prescribing for viral illness

SAY — Universal Prescribing Script: "Before prescribing I will check allergies, renal function, and pregnancy status. Cultures sent where appropriate. Starting empiric antibiotics per UK guidance. Review at 48–72h to narrow or switch IV to oral."

Step 1: Screen sepsis	NEWS2 + clinical judgement. If suspected: IV broad-spectrum within 1 hour.
Step 2: Safety checks	Allergies (penicillin) · eGFR · Pregnancy/breastfeeding · Recent antibiotic exposure
Step 3: Microbiology	Blood/urine/sputum cultures BEFORE antibiotics where possible. Do not delay if unstable.
Step 4: Stewardship	Review at 48–72h — narrow to cultures · stop if excluded · switch IV→oral when stable

SEPSIS SIX — Within 1 Hour

Do NOT delay in: Sepsis · Bacterial meningitis · Neutropenic sepsis · Septic arthritis · Severe pneumonia

#	Action	Rationale
1	Oxygen	Maintain SpO_2 >94%
2	Blood cultures	Before antibiotics where possible
3	IV Antibiotics	Broad-spectrum, IMMEDIATE
4	IV Fluids 500ml bolus	Assess response
5	Lactate measurement	Identifies tissue hypoperfusion
6	Urine output monitoring	Target >0.5 mL/kg/hr

High-Yield Infections — First-Line & Allergy Alternatives

Infection	First Line	Penicillin Allergy Alt	Duration/Notes
CAP (mild-mod)	Amoxicillin	Doxycycline or Clarithromycin	5 days
CAP (severe)	Co-amoxiclav + Clarithromycin IV	Discuss microbiology	Per specialist

Infection	First Line	Penicillin Allergy Alt	Duration/Notes
HAP	Piperacillin-Tazobactam IV	Microbiology advice	Local resistance patterns
Meningitis	Ceftriaxone IV (immediately)	Specialist regimen	+ Dexamethasone · Add Amoxicillin if >50/immunocomp (Listeria)
UTI (uncomplicated)	Nitrofurantoin (eGFR ≥45)	Trimethoprim	5 days · avoid fluoroquinolones
UTI (pregnancy)	Nitrofurantoin (avoid near term)	Cephalexin	7 days · avoid trimethoprim 1st trimester
Pyelonephritis (stable)	Ciprofloxacin oral		7 days
Pyelonephritis (unwell)	Ceftriaxone or Co-amoxiclav IV		Reassess 48–72h
Cellulitis	Flucloxacillin (oral if mild, IV if severe)	Clarithromycin or Doxycycline	Mark erythema border + reassess 24–48h
Sepsis (unknown source)	Piperacillin-Tazobactam IV	Microbiology advice	+Gentamicin if severe · +Vancomycin if MRSA risk
Neutropenic sepsis	Piperacillin-Tazobactam IV	+Vancomycin (line/instability)	EMERGENCY — start within 1 hour
PID	Ceftriaxone IM stat + Doxycycline + Metronidazole oral		14 days total
Septic arthritis	Flucloxacillin IV	+Vancomycin (MRSA) · +Ceftriaxone (GC)	URGENT joint aspiration before ABx if possible
Diabetic foot (mild)	Co-amoxiclav oral		Check circulation + neuropathy
Diabetic foot (severe)	Piperacillin-Tazobactam IV		Check for osteomyelitis + vascular review
Intra-abdominal	Piperacillin-Tazobactam	Ceftriaxone + Metronidazole	Source control ESSENTIAL
Cholangitis	Piperacillin-Tazobactam	Ceftriaxone + Metronidazole	Urgent ERCP for biliary drainage
Gonorrhoea	Ceftriaxone IM single dose		+Doxycycline if chlamydia not excluded
C. difficile	Oral Vancomycin ×10 days		Stop unnecessary antibiotics — essential

CAUTION — Penicillin Allergy · MRSA Risk · Do NOT Prescribe

Penicillin Allergy Clarification: "Was it a rash, swelling, or difficulty breathing?" — rash ≠ anaphylaxis. Confirm before substituting.

MRSA Risk Factors → Consider Vancomycin: Previous MRSA infection · nursing home resident · recent hospitalisation (<3 months) · haemodialysis · chronic wounds

Actions: Microbiology advice · add Vancomycin · monitor levels · isolate (contact precautions) · review at 48h cultures

DO NOT Prescribe Antibiotics For:

Viral URTI (reassure + symptom management) · Acute viral bronchitis (safety-net, review if no improvement 3 weeks) · Influenza (use antivirals if indicated) · Viral diarrhoea (ORS, investigate if bloody/prolonged) · Asymptomatic bacteriuria (treat only in pregnancy or pre-urological procedure)

Prescribing for viral illness = stewardship fail.

C. Diff Risk: Clindamycin (very high — avoid) · Cephalosporins (high) · Fluoroquinolones (high — epidemic strains) · Co-amoxiclav (moderate-high)

Top 10 Antibiotics for PLAB 2

Antibiotic (Class)	Key Use	Notes
Amoxicillin (aminopenicillin)	Mild CAP · otitis media · sinusitis	Oral / IV
Flucloxacillin (pen-resistant)	Cellulitis · septic arthritis (empiric)	Oral mild / IV severe
Co-amoxiclav (BL+inhibitor)	Diabetic foot · mild intra-abdominal	Moderate infections
Clarithromycin (macrolide)	Penicillin allergy CAP · atypical cover	QT prolongation caution
Doxycycline (tetracycline)	PID · pen allergy · atypicals	Avoid in pregnancy
Metronidazole (nitroimidazole)	Anaerobic cover · PID · C. diff (2nd line)	Oral or IV
Nitrofurantoin	Uncomplicated UTI (eGFR ≥45)	Avoid eGFR <45 · avoid near term
Ceftriaxone (3rd gen ceph)	Meningitis · septic arthritis · PID	IV · do not delay
Piperacillin-Tazobactam	Sepsis · HAP · neutropenic sepsis	IV · broad-spectrum
Vancomycin (glycopeptide)	MRSA · neutropenic sepsis · C. diff (oral)	Monitor levels · renal check

IV to Oral Switch — Criteria (48–72 Hours)

Switch Criteria	Safety Checks Before Switching
Clinical improvement noted	Record switch decision in notes
Afebrile for at least 24 hours	Confirm oral route bioavailability
Haemodynamically stable	Check drug-drug interactions for oral agent
Able to tolerate oral medication	Ensure appropriate oral dose (may differ from IV)
Infection source controlled	Communicate plan to nursing staff

Examiner Checklist

Prescribing Safety ✓	Stewardship ✓
✓ Sepsis recognised + antibiotics <1h	✓ 48–72h review plan stated
✓ Allergy check first	✓ IV to oral switch criteria known
✓ Renal function (eGFR) checked	✓ Not prescribing for viral illness
✓ Pregnancy status checked	✓ Indication documented
✓ Correct antibiotic for infection site	✓ Duration stated
✓ Allergy alternative known	✓ Cultures sent before antibiotics
✓ MRSA risk assessed	✓ C. diff risk considered
✓ Meningitis: no delay for CT/LP	✓ Source control (abdominal/joint)

Final Exam Mantra

Sepsis Six within 1 hour: O_2 · cultures · IV ABx · fluids · lactate · urine output
Universal checks: Allergy · eGFR · Pregnancy · Recent ABx exposure · Local guidelines
Meningitis + neutropenic sepsis + septic arthritis = DO NOT DELAY antibiotics
Stewardship: Review 48–72h · narrow to cultures · IV→oral when stable · stop if viral/excluded
Never prescribe for: viral URTI · viral bronchitis · asymptomatic bacteriuria (non-pregnant)

Allergy first every station always	Sepsis 1 hour do not delay	Meningitis now do not wait for CT/LP	Nitrofurantoin UTI eGFR ≥45 only	Ceftriaxone meningitis/septic arthritis
Pip-Tazo sepsis/HAP/neutropenic	IV-oral at 48-72h stewardship switch	Viral = no ABx stewardship tested	MRSA = Vancomycin check levels	Source control abscess/abdominal/joint

Appendix 2D · NORMAL VALUES & LABORATORY REFERENCE RANGES

UK/NHS ranges, SI units · Critical Values · Haematology · Biochemistry · ABG · ECG · Paediatric Vital Signs

Focus on critical values and common station abnormalities — not memorising every range

Critical Values — Automatic Escalation

Any critical value = escalate immediately: "This is a critical abnormality and I would escalate immediately to a senior doctor/ICU team."

Test	Critical Value	Why It Matters
Potassium	<2.5 or >6.5 mmol/L	Fatal arrhythmias
Sodium	<120 or >155 mmol/L	Seizure, coma
Glucose	<3 or >25 mmol/L	Hypoglycaemia, DKA/HHS
Lactate	>4 mmol/L	Severe sepsis / shock
Arterial pH	<7.2 or >7.55	Severe metabolic disturbance
Platelets	<20 $\times 10^9$/L	Spontaneous bleeding risk
Neutrophils	<0.5 $\times 10^9$/L	Neutropenic sepsis risk
Haemoglobin	<70 g/L	Transfusion threshold
PaO_2	<8 kPa (room air)	Respiratory failure
$PaCO_2$	>6.5 kPa + acidosis	Type 2 respiratory failure

Memory Shortcut: K · Na · Glucose · Lactate · pH · Hb · Neutrophils — the most exam-relevant dangerous values

Haematology · Biochemistry Reference Ranges

Test	Normal Range	Interpretation
Haemoglobin	M 130–170 g/L · F 115–155 g/L	Anaemia vs polycythaemia
WCC	4–11 $\times 10^9$/L	Infection / inflammation
Neutrophils	2–7.5 $\times 10^9$/L	Bacterial infection
Platelets	150–400 $\times 10^9$/L	Bleeding / thrombosis
MCV	80–100 fL	Microcytic vs macrocytic
INR	0.9–1.2	Warfarin monitoring
APTT	26–36 sec	Heparin / clotting

Test	Normal Range	Clinical Note
Sodium	135–145 mmol/L	Fluid balance
Potassium	3.5–5.0 mmol/L	Cardiac rhythm
Urea	2.5–7.0 mmol/L	Hydration / renal
Creatinine	60–110 μmol/L	Kidney function
eGFR	>90	Renal health
Glucose (fasting)	3.9–5.5 mmol/L	Diabetes
CRP	<5 mg/L	Inflammation
Lactate	<2 mmol/L	Tissue hypoxia
Calcium (corrected)	2.2–2.6 mmol/L	Bone / endocrine
Albumin	35–50 g/L	Nutrition / liver
ALT	10–50 U/L	Liver injury
ALP	30–130 U/L	Bone / liver
Bilirubin	<21 μmol/L	Jaundice

OSCE Tips: Low Hb + low MCV = iron deficiency · High MCV = B12/folate or alcohol · Corrected Ca = Ca + 0.02 × (40 − albumin)

ABG Normal Values · ECG Normal Values

ABG Parameter / ECG Parameter	Normal Range
pH	7.35–7.45
PaO_2	11–13 kPa
$PaCO_2$	4.7–6.0 kPa
HCO_3^-	22–26 mmol/L
Base excess	−2 to +2
Lactate	<2 mmol/L
Heart rate	60–100 bpm
PR interval	120–200 ms
QRS duration	<120 ms
QTc	<440 ms (M) · <460 ms (F)

Dangerous ECG Findings:
ST elevation = STEMI · Peaked T waves = Hyperkalaemia · U waves = Hypokalaemia · Wide QRS = Ventricular rhythm

ABG 5-Step PLAB Method: 1. pH 2. $PaCO_2$ 3. HCO_3^- 4. Respiratory vs metabolic 5. Oxygenation

Pregnancy Lab Changes · Paediatric Vital Signs

Pregnancy: Test	Expected Change
Haemoglobin	↓ (often 100–120 g/L) — physiological haemodilution
WCC	↑ (up to 15)
Platelets	Slight ↓
Urea & creatinine	↓
ALP	↑ (placental production)
Albumin	↓
TSH	Slight ↓ first trimester

Pregnancy tip: Hb of 105 g/L in pregnancy may be normal. Always interpret in clinical context.

Age	HR (bpm)	RR (/min)	SBP (mmHg)
Neonate	120–160	30–60	60–80
Infant	110–150	25–50	70–100
Toddler	90–140	20–35	80–110
School child	70–110	15–25	90–120
Adolescent	60–100	12–20	100–130

Paediatric Red Flags:
Temperature >38°C in <3 months = EMERGENCY — escalate immediately
Capillary refill >3 sec = Concerning — assess circulation · Neonatal glucose <2.6 mmol/L = Hypoglycaemia — treat immediately

Most Common PLAB 2 Lab Abnormalities · Escalation Phrase

#	Abnormality	Key Test(s)
1	Hyperkalaemia	K+, ECG
2	Sepsis lactate elevation	Lactate, VBG
3	DKA glucose + ketones	Glucose, VBG, ketones

#	Abnormality	Key Test(s)
4	Anaemia (low Hb)	FBC, MCV
5	AKI (raised creatinine)	Creatinine, U&E, eGFR
6	Hyponatraemia	Sodium, osmolality

SAY — OSCE Escalation Phrase: "This result is concerning and could indicate a serious condition. I would escalate immediately to my senior and initiate appropriate management."
Demonstrates: Clinical safety · Situational awareness · Team escalation

Final Exam Mantra

Critical Values: K <2.5/>6.5 · Na <120/>155 · Glucose <3/>25 · Lactate >4 · pH <7.2/>7.55 · Platelets <20 · Neutrophils <0.5 · Hb <70 · PaO_2 <8 kPa · $PaCO_2$ >6.5 + acidosis

Top 6 Abnormalities: Hyperkalaemia · Sepsis lactate · DKA · Anaemia · AKI · Hyponatraemia

Pregnancy changes: Hb ↓ (100–120 normal) · WCC ↑ · ALP ↑ · Albumin ↓ · Urea/creatinine ↓ · TSH slight ↓ first trimester

Paediatric red flags: Temp >38°C in <3 months = emergency · CRT >3 sec · Neonatal glucose <2.6

K+ critical <2.5 or >6.5 mmol/L	Na+ critical <120 or >155 mmol/L	Glucose critical <3 or >25 mmol/L	Lactate >4 ICU escalation	pH <7.2 >7.55 = escalate
Hb <70 transfusion threshold	PaO2 <8 kPa respiratory failure	Neonate temp >38 emergency escalate	CRT >3 sec assess circulation	Pregnancy Hb 100-120 may be normal

Appendix 2E · PRESCRIBING SAFETY MASTER REFERENCE

Top Prescribing Traps · High-Risk Drug Anchors · Universal Pre-Prescribing Checklist

AMaC (A. Mansour and Colleagues) · PLAB 2 Master Series · Volume 2 Reference

Three Prescribing Fails That End Stations Immediately:

1. **Methotrexate prescribed DAILY instead of ONCE WEEKLY — potentially fatal**
2. **Insulin written as "u" or "U" instead of "units" — 10× dosing error risk**
3. **Prescribing despite a documented allergy — instant fail regardless of clinical context**

✓ Universal Pre-Prescribing Checklist — Run This Before Every Prescription

Before writing or verbalising ANY prescription, run ACID-ID:

A = Allergies confirmed (ask + check chart) · C = Correct indication (why this drug, now?) · I = Indication and dose correct for this patient

D = Drug interactions checked · I = Individual factors (renal function, pregnancy, age, weight) · D = Document + explain to patient

"Before I prescribe, I would confirm there are no allergies, check the indication and dose, review renal function, check for interactions, and counsel the patient."

Step	Check	What to Ask	Fail if Missed
1	Allergy	"Any drug allergies or reactions?"	Yes — instant fail
2	Indication	"Why is this drug needed now?"	Often — unsafe prescribing
3	Dose + frequency	"Is this the correct dose, route, frequency?"	Yes — especially MTX/insulin
4	Renal function	"What is the eGFR/creatinine?"	Often — dose adjustment needed
5	Interactions	"What else is the patient taking?"	Common — warfarin + antibiotics
6	Special populations	Pregnancy · elderly · weight-based?	Often — contraindications
7	Pregnancy status	"Could she be pregnant? Test — do not assume."	Yes — test before prescribing in any woman of childbearing age
8	Decimal check	"0.1 or 1.0? Never a trailing zero."	Sometimes — 10× error risk
9	Sign + document	"Signed, dated, indication documented"	Yes — unsigned = invalid

Top Prescribing Traps — Wrong vs Correct

Drug / Situation	Common Wrong Answer	Correct Answer	Why It Matters
Methotrexate	"1mg daily"	"7.5mg ONCE WEEKLY — same day each week"	Daily = potentially fatal bone marrow suppression
Insulin	"10u" or "10U"	"10 units" — written in full always	"u" misread as "0" = 10× overdose
Warfarin + antibiotics	No monitoring plan	"Check INR in 48–72 hours — antibiotics raise INR"	Unmonitored warfarin = bleeding risk
Gentamicin	Fixed dose	"Weight-based: 5mg/kg ideal body weight · check levels"	Renal toxicity + ototoxicity if underdosed or overdosed
Opioids	No laxatives prescribed	"Always co-prescribe laxatives — constipation universal"	Opioid-induced constipation = automatic oversight fail
NSAIDs + CKD	Prescribe as normal	"Contraindicated in CKD — use paracetamol instead"	Nephrotoxic — AKI risk
NSAIDs + 3rd trimester	Prescribe as normal	"Contraindicated in 3rd trimester — premature ductus closure"	Fetal harm
Warfarin — major bleed	"Give Vitamin K only"	"PCC (Beriplex) immediately PLUS IV Vitamin K"	Vitamin K alone too slow for life-threatening bleed
ACE inhibitor + sick day	Continue as normal	"STOP if vomiting/diarrhoea/dehydrated — restart when eating"	AKI risk when dehydrated
Lithium — toxicity	Reassure and continue	"STOP lithium — check levels urgently — TAC: tremor, ataxia, confusion"	Narrow therapeutic index — toxicity life-threatening
Steroid — stopping	"Stop immediately"	"Taper slowly — never stop abruptly if >3 weeks"	Adrenal crisis risk
IV fluids — hyponatraemia	Correct rapidly	"Correct slowly — max 8–10 mmol/L per 24 hours"	Rapid correction = central pontine myelinolysis (CPM)
Hypoglycaemia treatment	"Give insulin"	"Fast-acting glucose now — NEVER give more insulin"	Insulin in hypoglycaemia = fatal

Drug / Situation	Common Wrong Answer	Correct Answer	Why It Matters
Penicillin allergy — cephalosporin	Avoid all cephalosporins	"Cross-reactivity ~1–2% — clarify reaction type first"	"I had a rash" ≠ anaphylaxis — may be safe
Digoxin + renal impairment	Standard dose	"Reduce dose — check eGFR — renally cleared"	Accumulation = toxicity: yellow vision, arrhythmia
Metformin + AKI/contrast	Continue	"STOP before contrast — hold if AKI or eGFR <30"	Lactic acidosis risk
Aminophylline/theophylline	No monitoring	"Check levels — narrow therapeutic index — interactions"	Toxicity: seizures, arrhythmias
Oxygen — COPD	"Give 15L via NRB mask"	"Target 88–92% in COPD — Venturi 28% or 24%"	High-flow oxygen in COPD = hypercapnic drive suppression
Hypoglycaemia threshold	Unclear / not defined	"<4 mmol/L = hypoglycaemia — <3 = severe — treat immediately"	Examiners expect precise threshold
VRIII — Variable Rate Insulin	Start without glucose check	"Check glucose before VRIII — run alongside 5% glucose or 0.9% NaCl"	VRIII without glucose context = hypoglycaemia risk

SADMAN — Sick-Day Rules · Stop These When Unwell

SADMAN: drugs to STOP if patient is vomiting, diarrhoea, or severely dehydrated:
S = Sulphonylureas (glibenclamide, gliclazide) · A = ACE inhibitors · D = Diuretics · M = Metformin · A = ARBs · N = NSAIDs
"These drugs become dangerous when the patient is dehydrated. Stop them and restart when eating and drinking normally."
Restart instruction: "Restart once you are eating and drinking normally for 24–48 hours."

Diabetes Prescribing Safety · VRIII · Hypoglycaemia

Hypoglycaemia Thresholds — Must Know Exactly:
<4.0 mmol/L = Hypoglycaemia — treat immediately
<3.0 mmol/L = Severe hypoglycaemia — IV glucose / glucagon
Treatment: fast-acting glucose (Lucozade 150mL / 3-4 glucose tabs / Glucogel) · recheck in 15 minutes · if unconscious: IV 10% glucose 200mL or IM glucagon 1mg
NEVER give more insulin · NEVER give slow-release carbohydrate alone first

VRIII Safety Check	Rule
Before starting VRIII	Check blood glucose — document baseline
Run alongside	0.9% NaCl with KCl or 5% glucose — NEVER run VRIII alone

VRIII Safety Check	Rule
Check glucose	Hourly initially · 2-hourly when stable
If glucose <6 on VRIII	Reduce rate · give glucose supplement
Never	Start VRIII without a glucose source running alongside
SADMAN drugs	STOP metformin + sulphonylureas when on VRIII
Sick-day DKA triggers	Glucose >11 + ketones >3 + acidosis → DKA pathway

Local Anaesthetic Safety · Lidocaine Toxicity

Before injecting local anaesthetic — ALWAYS:
1. Confirm allergy (lidocaine/amide group) · 2. Aspirate before injecting — blood in syringe = intravascular = STOP
3. Use minimum effective dose · 4. Know maximum dose: lidocaine 3mg/kg (plain) · 7mg/kg (with adrenaline)

Lidocaine Toxicity — LAST mnemonic:
L = Lightheadedness + tinnitus (early warning) · A = Arrhythmia (severe) · S = Seizures · T = Toxicity = STOP + call for help + Intralipid 20%
"If I notice tinnitus or dizziness during injection I would STOP immediately, call for help, and prepare for advanced resuscitation."

Electrolyte · Fluid Safety · Critical Corrections

Electrolyte Issue	Critical Rule	Why
Hyponatraemia	NEVER correct faster than 8–10 mmol/L per 24 hours	Rapid correction = Central Pontine Myelinolysis (CPM) = irreversible brainstem demyelination
Hyperkalaemia >6.5	ECG first — calcium gluconate if peaked T waves — then insulin/dextrose	Peaked T waves = imminent arrhythmia — calcium gluconate membrane-stabilises within minutes
Hypokalaemia <2.5	Replace IV if <2.5 or symptomatic — NEVER bolus — max 20 mmol/hour	Bolus potassium = cardiac arrest
IV fluids + heart failure	Caution — restrict volume — consider furosemide cover	Fluid overload worsens pulmonary oedema
IV fluids + CKD	Use 0.9% NaCl cautiously — avoid K+ containing fluids if hyperkalaemic	Renal impairment = electrolyte retention risk
Magnesium	Check Mg in hypokalaemia refractory to K+ replacement	Hypomagnesaemia prevents K+ correction

Psychiatry Drug Safety

Drug	Key Safety Points
SSRIs	Increased suicide risk in first 2 weeks especially in under-25s — review early — serotonin syndrome if combined with MAOIs/tramadol — never stop abruptly — taper over 4 weeks
Lithium	TAC toxicity: Tremor (coarse) · Ataxia · Confusion — check levels urgently if any symptoms — STOP and seek help — narrow therapeutic index 0.4–1.0 mmol/L
Antipsychotics	NMS (fever + rigidity + confusion + autonomic instability) = STOP + ICU — QT prolongation (check ECG) — metabolic syndrome monitoring (weight, glucose, lipids)
Benzodiazepines	Dependence risk — never prescribe long-term — 2–4 weeks maximum — withdrawal seizures if stopped abruptly — assess capacity before prescribing in addiction context
MAOIs	Serotonin syndrome with SSRIs/tramadol/pethidine — hypertensive crisis with tyramine-rich foods — rare in PLAB 2 but deadly interaction — always ask about MAOI use

SAY — What to Say When You Don't Know — Recovery Scripts

The silence that fails stations is never about not knowing. It is about not knowing what to say when you don't know.
These scripts keep you safe, sound professional, and demonstrate the most important competency in PLAB 2: knowing your limits.

Situation	What to Say — Word for Word
You don't know the diagnosis	"I don't have a clear diagnosis at this point. My priority is to ensure this patient is safe. I would apply ABCDE, take a full history, and escalate to my senior for review."
You don't know the dose	"I know the correct drug in this situation. For the precise dose I would check the BNF and confirm with my senior before prescribing — I would not guess a dose."
You don't know the drug name	"I would treat this condition with an antibiotic targeting [gram positive/gram negative] organisms — I would confirm the specific agent with the BNF and consult microbiology if needed."
You freeze mid-station	"I'm going to take 10 seconds to organise my thoughts — thank you for your patience." (pause, breathe, continue with ICE or ABCDE as anchor)
Examiner asks a question you can't answer	"That's a really important point. I'm not certain of the exact answer, but I know I would escalate this to my senior and look it up in the BNF/guidelines before acting."
Patient asks something clinical you don't know	"That's a very good question. I want to give you accurate information rather than guess — I will look that up and come back to you, or I can arrange for a specialist to discuss it with you."

Situation	What to Say — Word for Word
You realise mid-station you made an error	"I want to correct something I said earlier — I said [X] but the correct answer is [Y]. I apologise for any confusion. Patient safety is my priority and I want to make sure I give you accurate information."
Station feels like it's going wrong	Return to ICE: "Can I just check — what was your main concern today?" Return to safety-net: "Have I answered your main question?" These anchors recover most stations.

Golden Rule for Uncertainty: "I don't know the exact answer, but I know how to keep this patient safe" is a passing answer in PLAB 2. Silence is not.

Examiners do not expect perfection. They expect safety, honesty, and appropriate escalation. These three scripts deliver all three.

Final Prescribing Mantra

Before every prescription: ACID-ID — Allergy · Correct indication · Indication+dose · Drug interactions · Individual factors · Document

MTX = ONCE WEEKLY · Insulin = "units" in full · Warfarin bleed = PCC + Vit K · SADMAN = stop when unwell

Hypo = <4 mmol/L · VRIII = check glucose first + run alongside glucose · Sodium = correct slowly (CPM risk)

Lidocaine = aspirate first · LAST toxicity = Lightheadedness, Arrhythmia, Seizures · Intralipid 20% reversal

Don't know the dose? Check BNF + escalate. Don't know the diagnosis? ABCDE + escalate. Never guess. Never silence.

Gold Closing — Any Prescribing Station:

"Allergies confirmed. Indication clear. Dose and frequency correct. Renal function checked. Interactions reviewed. Patient counselled with teach-back. Monitoring arranged. Documented clearly."

ACID-ID always before every prescription	**MTX once weekly** never daily = fatal	**Insulin = units** never u or U	**Hypo = <4 mmol/L** severe = <3 treat now	**VRIII + glucose** never run alone
SADMAN sick-day stop when dehydrated	**Sodium slow** CPM if corrected fast	**Lidocaine LAST** aspirate before injecting	**PCC + Vit K** warfarin major bleed	**Don't know = escalate** never silence or guess

Appendix 2F · Instant Fail Triggers Quick Reminder

Condensed reference · Full version in Volume 1 (App 1B)

True Failure Causes: Safety breach · Consent violation · Suicide mismanagement · Safeguarding failure · Major prescribing error · Professionalism lapse

#	Category	Key Instant Fail Triggers
1	Consent & Capacity	No consent · No chaperone (intimate exam) · Continue after refusal · Ignore capacity issues
2	Clinical Danger	Send high-risk chest pain home · Miss cauda equina · No ABCDE in collapse · No O_2 in hypoxia
3	Prescribing	Prescribe despite allergy · 10× dose error · No allergy check · Contraindicated in pregnancy
4	Safeguarding	Ignore child protection · Ignore abuse disclosure · Promise secrecy
5	Suicide & MH	No suicide screen when indicated · Miss intent/plan · Discharge high-risk without safety plan
6	Ethics	Breach confidentiality · Lie to patient · Falsify documentation
7	Bad News	No warning shot · Never says "cancer" clearly · Continue while patient is crying

SAFE Rule: Safety first · Ask ICE + assess risk · Flag emergencies · Explain clearly + safety-net

Subtle Fatal Combinations (Tier 2):
Poor empathy + unsafe discharge · No ICE + imposed plan · No suicide screen + false reassurance

Appendix 2G · Station Micro-Summary Quick Reminder

Condensed reference · Full version in Volume 1 (App 1D)

Top 5 Must-Say Phrases:
ICE: "What do you think? Any worries? What were you hoping for?"
Safety-Net: "Return if symptoms worsen, new symptoms appear, or you're worried."
Escalate: "I would discuss this with my senior."
Empathy: "That sounds really difficult."
SDM: "Some prefer X, others Y — what are your thoughts?"

Emergency Must-Says:
"I am concerned about a potentially serious condition."
"I would start an ABCDE assessment."
"I would call for senior help."
"I would reassess after intervention."
"I would document and hand over clearly."

H	HISTORY	Hello · ICE · Set agenda · Take history (SOCRATES) · Other background · Reflect · Your safety-net
S	SAFE PLAN	Summarise safety · Assess · Formulate 5Ps · Explain SDM · Liaise/escalate · Arrange follow-up · Never forget safety-net
B	BREAKDOWN	Begin permission · Results · Explain simply · Assess understanding · Keep ICE · Discuss options · Offer written info · Wonder about questions · Next steps
B	BRIDGE	Build rapport · Recognise emotion · ICE deep dive · Do not argue, bridge · Give info gently · Explore options collaboratively

2-Minute Flow: Before: hygiene + observe · First 30s: introduce + ICE · Middle: signpost + template + empathy + verbalise · End: SDM + safety-net + close + document
Emergency Override: Patient unstable → STOP. Switch to ABCDE. Call for help. Resume only when safe.

MASTER GLOSSARY · ABBREVIATIONS

Abbrev	Meaning	Abbrev	Meaning
ACS	Acute Coronary Syndrome	**LARC**	Long-Acting Reversible Contraception
ADRT	Advance Decision to Refuse Treatment	**LMP**	Last Menstrual Period
AFI	Amniotic Fluid Index	**LMWH**	Low Molecular Weight Heparin
AHT	Abusive Head Trauma	**LNG**	Levonorgestrel
AKI	Acute Kidney Injury	**LNG-IUS**	Levonorgestrel Intrauterine System
AMH	Anti-Mullerian Hormone	**LP**	Lumbar Puncture
AMTS	Abbreviated Mental Test Score	**LPA**	Lasting Power of Attorney
ANC	Antenatal Care	**MART**	Maintenance & Reliever Therapy
APS	Antiphospholipid Syndrome	**MDT**	Multidisciplinary Team
AVPU	Alert, Voice, Pain, Unresponsive	**MHA**	Mental Health Act
BNF	British National Formulary	**MHP**	Major Haemorrhage Protocol
BPP	Biophysical Profile	**MMR**	Measles, Mumps & Rubella
CAP	Community-Acquired Pneumonia	**MRC**	Medical Research Council scale
CBT	Cognitive Behavioural Therapy	**MRSA**	Meticillin-Resistant Staphylococcus aureus
CGA	Comprehensive Geriatric Assessment	**MTX**	Methotrexate
CICV	Cannot Intubate, Cannot Ventilate	**NAI**	Non-Accidental Injury
CKD	Chronic Kidney Disease	**NBM**	Nil By Mouth
COC	Combined Oral Contraceptive	**NEWS2**	National Early Warning Score 2
COCP	Combined Oral Contraceptive Pill	**NIV**	Non-Invasive Ventilation
COPD	Chronic Obstructive Pulmonary Disease	**NRT**	Nicotine Replacement Therapy
CPM	Central Pontine Myelinolysis	**NTD**	Neural Tube Defect
CRAO	Central Retinal Artery Occlusion	**PCC**	Prothrombin Complex Concentrate
CRT	Capillary Refill Time	**PCI**	Percutaneous Coronary Intervention
CTG	Cardiotocography	**PCV**	Packed Cell Volume
CTPA	CT Pulmonary Angiogram	**PE**	Pulmonary Embolism
DKA	Diabetic Ketoacidosis	**PEA**	Pulseless Electrical Activity
DNACPR	Do Not Attempt Cardiopulmonary Resuscitation	**PHQ-9**	Patient Health Questionnaire-9
DPI	Dry Powder Inhaler	**PID**	Pelvic Inflammatory Disease
DVLA	Driver & Vehicle Licensing Agency	**PLAB**	Professional & Linguistic Assessments Board
DVT	Deep Vein Thrombosis	**POP**	Progestogen-Only Pill

EBL	Estimated Blood Loss	**PPH**	Postpartum Haemorrhage
EEG	Electroencephalogram	**PPI**	Proton Pump Inhibitor
EPDS	Edinburgh Postnatal Depression Scale	**PSV**	Public Service Vehicle
ERPC	Evacuation of Retained Products of Conception	**QRISK3**	QRISK3 cardiovascular risk score
FGM	Female Genital Mutilation	**RAPD**	Relative Afferent Pupillary Defect
FII	Fabricated or Induced Illness	**RFM**	Reduced Fetal Movements
FRIII	Fixed Rate Intravenous Insulin Infusion	**ROSC**	Return of Spontaneous Circulation
FSH	Follicle-Stimulating Hormone	**RSI**	Rapid Sequence Induction
FSRH	Faculty of Sexual & Reproductive Healthcare	**RUQ**	Right Upper Quadrant
FTU	Fingertip Unit	**SABA**	Short-Acting Beta-Agonist
GAD-7	Generalised Anxiety Disorder scale-7	**SARC**	Sexual Assault Referral Centre
GCA	Giant Cell Arteritis	**SBP**	Systolic Blood Pressure
GDM	Gestational Diabetes Mellitus	**SGLT2**	Sodium-Glucose Cotransporter-2 inhibitor
GLP-1	Glucagon-Like Peptide-1 agonist	**SSRI**	Selective Serotonin Reuptake Inhibitor
GTN	Glyceryl Trinitrate	**STEMI**	ST-Elevation Myocardial Infarction
HAP	Hospital-Acquired Pneumonia	**SVC**	Superior Vena Cava
HGV	Heavy Goods Vehicle	**TCA**	Tricyclic Antidepressant
HHS	Hyperosmolar Hyperglycaemic State	**TLS**	Tumour Lysis Syndrome
HPV	Human Papillomavirus	**TRALI**	Transfusion-Related Acute Lung Injury
HRT	Hormone Replacement Therapy	**TVUSS**	Transvaginal Ultrasound Scan
HSG	Hysterosalpingogram	**TXA**	Tranexamic Acid
ICD	Implantable Cardioverter Defibrillator	**UKMEC**	UK Medical Eligibility Criteria
ICP	Intracranial Pressure	**UPA**	Ulipristal Acetate
ITP	Immune Thrombocytopenia	**UPSI**	Unprotected Sexual Intercourse
IUD	Intrauterine Device	**URTI**	Upper Respiratory Tract Infection
IUGR	Intrauterine Growth Restriction	**USS**	Ultrasound Scan
IUP	Intrauterine Pregnancy	**VA**	Visual Acuity
IUS	Intrauterine System	**VF**	Ventricular Fibrillation
IVF	In Vitro Fertilisation	**VRIII**	Variable Rate Intravenous Insulin Infusion
JVP	Jugular Venous Pressure	**VTE**	Venous Thromboembolism
LABA	Long-Acting Beta-Agonist		

www.ingramcontent.com/pod-product-compliance
Lightning Source LLC
LaVergne TN
LVHW010721061126
851857LV00014B/1296
9781066746729